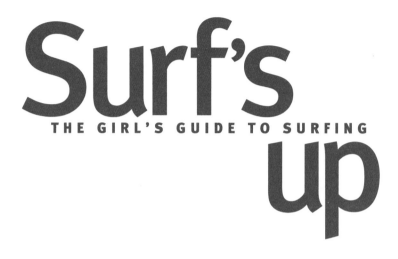

Surf's

THE GIRL'S GUIDE TO SURFING

up

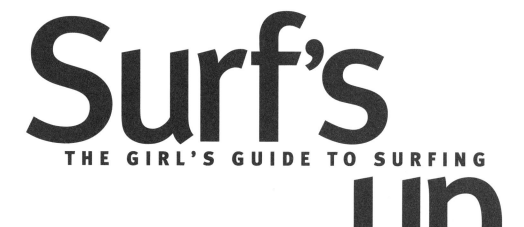

Surf's up

THE GIRL'S GUIDE TO SURFING

LOUISE SOUTHERDEN

BALLANTINE BOOKS ✳ **NEW YORK**

2005 Ballantine Books Trade Paperback Edition

Copyright © 2003, 2005 by Louise Southerden

Published in the United States by Ballantine Books, an imprint of The Random House Publishing Group, a division of Random House, Inc., New York.

Ballantine and colophon are registered trademarks of Random House, Inc.

Originally published in different form in Australia by Allen & Unwin in Crows Nest. NSW, in 2003.

Library of Congress Cataloging-in-Publication Data

Southerden, Louise.
Surf's up : the girl's guide to surfing / Louise Southerden.—1st American ed.
p.   cm.
ISBN 0-345-47661-1
1. Surfing for women.   I. Title.
GV840.S8S695 2005
797.3'2'08—dc22   2004057002

Printed in the United States of America

Ballantine books website address: www.ballantinebooks.com

9 8 7 6 5 4 3 2 1

For my dad, and our shared
love of the ocean

thanks

✻

A frangipani to the following people who helped in ways great and small: The surfer girls interviewed—Angie Gosch, Belinda Glynn, Esther Hamburger, Alison Aprhys, Loata Sanderson, Emy Tesoriero, Bethany Currin, Deborah Stoll, Anna Cooper, and Kaitlyn Margeson—for openly sharing their insights and experiences of the learning-to-surf curve. Janet Boyd, my Montauk, Long Island, friend, who helped so much with the research for this US edition; as did Jim Regan, who is truly the best friend a writer could ever have. Christine Schiedel for her beautifully creative design of the book. Izzy Tihanyi of Surf Diva Surf School, Karina and Erik Petroni, Bethany Hamilton and her manager Roy Hofstetter, John Radcliffe at Dripping Wet Surf Co., Penny Lane of Manly Surf School, Shawn Ambrose of Trixie Surfboards, and surf coaches Mary Setterholm, Priscilla-Anne Hensler, Anna Santoro, and Ross Phillips at Surf Schools International, for their input. Kirsten Tremlett for the surf stretches. Kathy Phillips of the Eastern Surfing Association, Marie Case at Board-Trac, Michael Gerard at Surfing America, Bryan Dickerson and Sunshine Makarow at *Surf Life for Women*, Tom Dugan at *Eastern Surf Magazine,* Todd Leetch at Girl in the Curl surf shop, and Nick at Hansen's Surfboards, for helping with the research. Layne Beachley for the inspiring foreword and for being such an upstanding role model for surfer girls everywhere. Pro surfers Rochelle Ballard, Serena Brooke, Kate Skarratt, Prue Jeffries, and Jodie Nelson, for their quotes and for giving women's surfing a higher profile than ever before. For assistance in researching the history of women's surfing, I thank Ray Moran of Manly Life Saving Club; Tina Graham of Warringah Library Local Studies Unit; *Girl in the Curl: A century of women in surfing* by Andrea Gabbard (Seal Press, Seattle, 2000); *The Glide: Longboarding and the renaissance of modern surfing*, edited by the late Chris Bystrom (Duranbah Press, Queensland, 1998); and *Blue Heaven: The Story of Australian Surfing* by Murray Walding (Hardie Grant Books, Victoria, 2003). Betty Leighton for permission to use one of the late Ray Leighton's photographs (page 8). Ocean & Earth for the Karlee Mackie images (Chapters 2 and 10). Rick Irons at Primedia for permission to use the *Surfer* magazine cover featuring Lisa Andersen (page 24). Photographers Neil Armstrong (Moonwalker), Joli, Simon Williams, Will Burgess, Jon Wellings, Jon

Steele, Josh Kimball, and Noah Hamilton, for their beautiful images. This US edition would not have happened without Marie Beard at Allen & Unwin. Heartfelt thanks too to my editor, Allison Dickens at Random House, who has been a joy to work with, on many levels. And finally warm, sunny thanks to you, the reader, for making the efforts of everyone mentioned here all the more worthwhile.

foreword

The ocean is constantly changing and is impossible to control, and yet, as surfers, we need a strong ability to read and understand it. We have to learn how to read the sandbanks, the currents, the movement of the swell. We have to understand the effects of the wind and swell and tidal changes on where and when waves break. We need to be able to determine how each wave breaks, how far out it's breaking, how far in, if it's a left or a right, if it's hollow or fat, fast or slow. Confused yet?

If you are, that's okay, because you're holding in your hands one of the most valuable tools a surfer girl could have. *Surf's Up: The Girl's Guide to Surfing* tackles everything you need to know both in and out of the water, saving you time, energy, and embarrassment!

I wish I had this book before making the trek down to Manly Beach in Sydney when I was learning. Intimidating guy surfers, a lack of skill, and little understanding of surfing etiquette were just some of the many hurdles I had to overcome, on my own, as a novice surfer. None of this stood in the way of my surfing passion, of course, and you shouldn't allow it to stand in your way either.

Surfing is a challenge, but that's why we love it, that's what makes it so special. Whenever I'm at the beach, my senses open as soon as my feet touch the sand. The fresh smell of salt air, the sound of the crashing swell, the soothing immersion in the water, the sight of dolphins playing and fish frenzying beneath my board. The world of surfing is just that—a whole new world waiting to be discovered by you. I hope the words of wisdom in the following pages help you in all ways to get out there and find your own special moments in the water.

Layne Beachley
Six-time world surfing champion
June 2004

author's note

Six months ago, I had the worst wipeout of my life. I was surfing at a beach break five hours north of Sydney with my friend Jim when I misjudged the takeoff on a set wave and went down with the lip. I didn't hit the bottom, but I hit the water so hard that my head bent too far forward, pinching my spinal cord and paralyzing me from the neck down. I had one thought: This is it.

Finally, after what seemed like a lifetime underwater, I floated to the surface face up and started calling for help. All I could do was float on my back and wait for the waves to wash me onto the beach. But Jim had seen my wipeout, and within minutes he and two other surfers were sliding me onto his longboard and carrying me to the beach; from there I was airlifted to a local base hospital and then to Sydney. It turned out that I was supremely lucky that day; my spinal cord was only bruised, not broken. I spent two weeks in the spinal unit of a Sydney hospital, and three months after that, getting the feeling and movement back in my arms and legs.

It might seem strange to start a learn-to-surf book with such a story, but I'm telling it to inspire you, not to scare you, because I think surfing actually saved my life. After a lifetime of wipeouts, I didn't panic when I was underwater for so long. I didn't lose consciousness or swallow any water. I knew to stay calm, relax as much as I could, and trust that the ocean would release me—and it did. Because I was relatively healthy and fit, my body healed itself quickly. Most important, being a surfer meant that I had the ocean for my rehabilitation—I spent all summer floating and then swimming in the ocean, gradually swimming farther out past the breaking waves to where I felt most at home. I even repaired my wetsuit (it had been cut off my body when I arrived in hospital) as part of my therapy. Stitch by stitch, I hand-sewed my life back together. Being a surfer may not make you immune to life's down times, but it can give you skills to ride them out.

Now, as I've been working on this completely revised edition of *Surf's Up*, tailor-made for American surfer girls, I'm rediscovering my love of surfing. Last Saturday I tried out my "new improved" wetsuit for the first time at one of my favorite surf beaches. The waves were overhead but full because of the high tide, and three of my friends were surfing, so I decided to paddle out to sit out the back with them. It took me a while to find the right moment (and the courage) to get through the shorebreak, but as soon as I started paddling it was like I'd never been away. After six months, it was reassuring to know it was all still there—my love of the ocean environment, feeling at home sitting on my board in deep water with other surfers, my sense of where the waves were and where it was "safe" to sit—and to feel a fresh appreciation for this incredible lifestyle we enjoy as surfers.

I've been reminded that no matter what level we surf at, what craft we ride, whether we surf standing up or kneeling or lying down, nothing beats that feeling of catching and riding a wave. I've been surfing a few times since that first paddle last week, and I realized something else each time I came home with wet hair and my board under my arm: I felt happy. From the very first time you set foot in the water with a surfboard, surfing begins to work its magic on you. I hope you enjoy *Surf's Up,* and may surfing bless your life in more ways than you can imagine.

June 2004

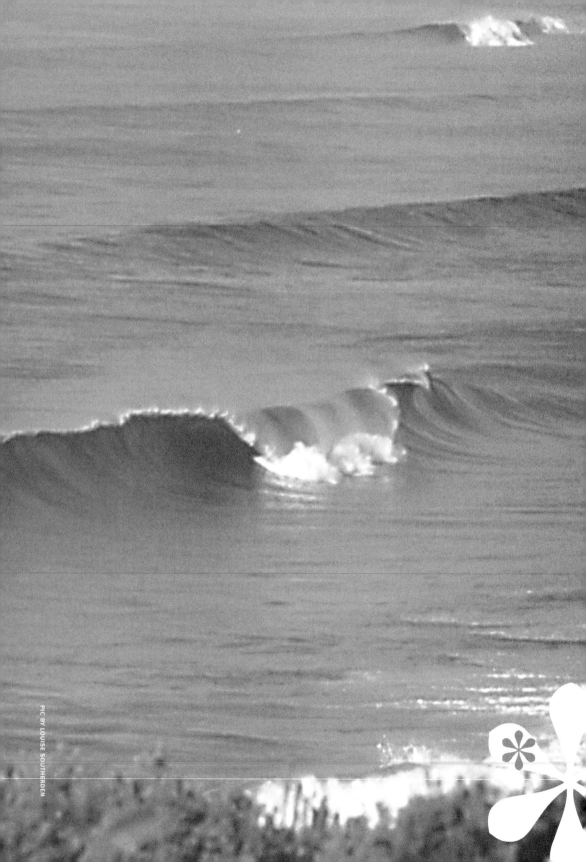

contents

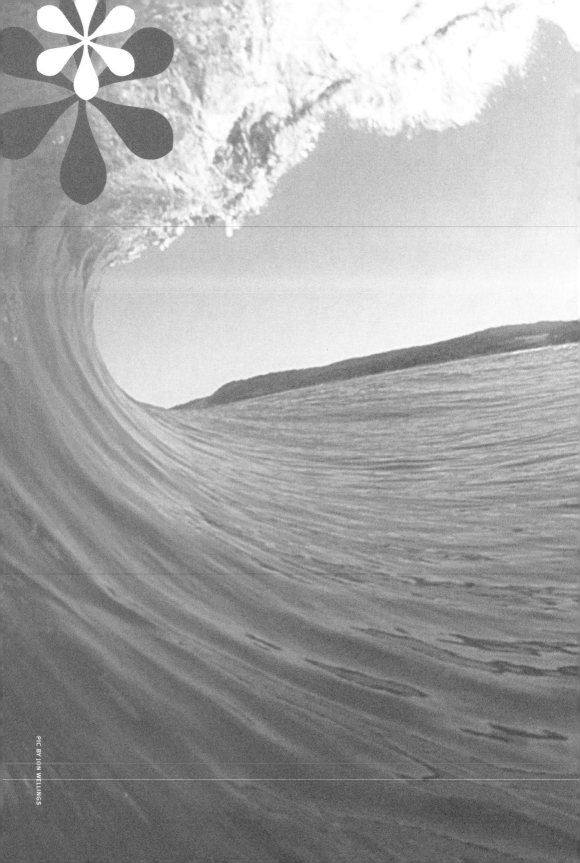

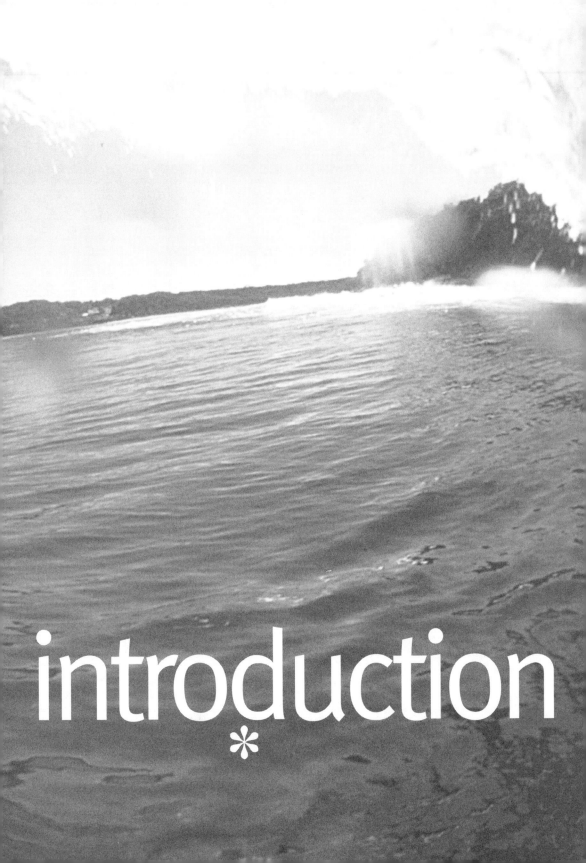

introduction

*

Y ou're about to be initiated into another world, a world of "dawn patrols" and "duck dives," "kooks" and "closeouts." You're going to be caught inside, barreled, and, one day, ripping it up. You can get there by yourself, but it's easier and more fun if you go with someone who knows the territory. That's where this book comes in, to keep you company and be your friend on the road to becoming a surfer. Read it at your own pace, ask it questions, and use it for moral support when the going gets tough. Surfing may be a solo activity, but it makes you part of a global community that stretches from coast to coast and across the oceans of this vast blue planet. Welcome to it.

My surfing life

When I learned to surf on Sydney's northern beaches almost fifteen years ago, girl surfers were a rare species. You couldn't go down to your local surf spot and check out the other girls in the water, because there weren't any. You couldn't watch a video of your favorite pro surfers, because no one made films of girls surfing back then. There were no women's surfing magazines, and none of the surf shops stocked women's gear. I had to wear a boy's wetsuit for the first year, until I managed to find one for girls—it was hot pink and blue (wetsuit manufacturers still clung to the antiquated notion that all girls adore wearing pink) and I cursed its conspicuousness when all I wanted to do was dissolve into the water so no one would see the blunders I was making.

And I was making plenty. I didn't kid myself that I had any natural talent, but the learn-to-surf process was made even harder by the fact that you had to teach yourself. The only consolation was that that's how everyone learned back then—there were no surf schools, surf lessons, or surf camps. The most you could hope for were surfing friends who, if you managed to catch them between the parking lot and the water's edge, might give you a piece of advice the way you'd toss hot fries to a seagull.

It was hard and lonely, but there was something about being the only girl out there that made me feel brave and special. On the rare occasions when I did see another surfing female, there was an instant camaraderie between us. Not only that, but we were free of the competitiveness that drove male surfers to outperform each other; we could just get out there and surf for the sheer fun of it.

Still, it was a long time before I actually felt like a surfer, partly because I felt so different from all the other surfers I knew. They were all guys for one thing; they surfed so fearlessly, and they looked like they'd been surfing since they were toddlers (whereas I'd started relatively late, when I was twenty-four). But they also wore their surfer image like a badge of honor, hanging out after surf sessions, smoking roll-your-owns and telling big-wave stories as they leaned against their old salt-encrusted station wagons.

Eventually, I don't know when exactly, I realized something: There are as many different ways to be a surfer as there are surfers themselves. It might sound obvious, given the huge range of people and surf craft out in the waves these days, but it was one of the most important lessons I ever learned because it marked the real beginning of my surfing life, the point at which I started creating my own relationship to surfing and the sea.

I've been surfing for a while now, and I can honestly say I love it as much as I ever have. Sometimes I think surfing has spoiled me—I have known such pure happiness in the ocean that few other experiences, places, or achievements can match it. I've surfed with dolphins, seen the sea lit by sunrises and studded with raindrops, been places I never would have been if I didn't surf. I feel younger, in body and mind, than I did before I started surfing. And it amazes me to think that, after all this time, checking the surf every morning is as much a part of my daily routine as brushing my teeth.

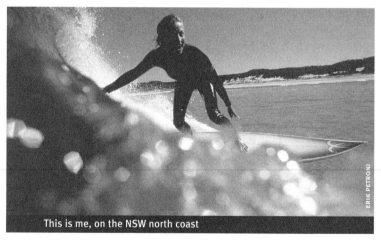
ERIK PETRONI

This is me, on the NSW north coast

It's an exciting time to be a surfer girl. Nevertheless, I'll always think of myself as a surfer first and a female surfer second. Maybe that's because my surfing life began at a time when girls who surfed were treated as inferior life forms. But I like to think it's also because, to me, surfing is a way of life that transcends gender, race, age, and any of the other barriers we put up between one another. When I lived in Japan, one of my Japanese girlfriends said to me, "When you're out in the ocean, it doesn't matter if you're a man or a woman; everyone's out there for their own reasons, doing their own thing." That's exactly how I feel. We're all just surfers, after all.

You can't learn to surf from a book!

That's true—but you're not going to. You're going to be out in the waves putting in your time like anyone else, making your own mistakes, learning things no one could have told you about the ocean and the waves and the way your surfboard responds when you move around on it. But there are advantages to having a learn-to-surf book by your side while you go through this learning process:

- It's patient: a book will never snap at you or make you feel stupid for reading the same bit over and over again.
- It's always there: a book is never too tired or too busy to answer your questions, so you can consult it when it suits you and when you've got a question, without having to wait for your next surf lesson.
- It's private: you can read up on things you might be embarrassed to ask about in front of other beginner surfers. Plus, it won't compare you to anyone else. When you're here, it's just you.
- You can travel at your own pace: you can go out and practice something as soon as you read it; you can read the whole book from cover to cover and go back to the bits you want to try; you can even skip over sections that aren't relevant to you (how many surf coaches let you ignore them like that?).
- It's girl-friendly: there are lots of girl-specific tips like how to find a bikini that will stay on in the surf and how to keep your hair in good condition.

What's inside

You probably can't wait to get started, so I'll keep this brief. Here's a map of the territory covered in the following pages:

Chapter 1: Looking back. It might seem weird to start a how-to book with a history of women's surfing—and you might want to skip over this section on your first read-through—but getting a glimpse of the long line of women surfers who have come before you can be really inspiring.

Chapter 2: Where to begin. Not sure where to start? This is the "Why are we here?" chapter. It includes ten reasons why you should learn to surf, a few skills you need before you embark on this big adventure, the pros and cons of surf lessons, and a few reservations (okay, fears) you might have about sharks, jellyfish stings, being hit by your surfboard, rips, and aggressive surfers. It also explains how surfing changes your body, if not your whole outlook on life.

Chapter 3: What you'll need. Now for the gritty details: what you need to go surfing, including how to choose the right surfboard, why long surfboards are better to learn on than shortboards, the costs involved, board-buying tips, what to wear in the water, and other essential ingredients such as leashes, wetsuits, wax, surfboard bags, sunscreen, and roof racks.

Chapter 4: Where to surf. Everything you need to know about how waves are formed; how they're affected by wind, tides, sand, and the shape of the beach; how to check the surf and decode weather reports so you can predict when waves are coming; and what kinds of waves you should be looking for.

Chapter 5: On the beach. All the last-minute pre-departure details including how to get changed in the parking lot (very important!), how to wax your surfboard, how to attach your leash to your board and, later, to your ankle (and how to know which ankle), pre-surf stretches, and what to take to the beach with you.

Chapter 6: Getting out there. Enough preparation already, let's do it! This chapter covers everything you need to get from the water's edge to sitting on your board out past the whitewater, waiting for your first wave, the art of paddling a surfboard, how to lie and sit on your board, and techniques to get you through the whitewater.

Chapter 7: How to catch waves. Now for the big one: how to catch broken waves (foam or whitewater), and then how to catch breaking (green) waves; the three keys to standing up; and how to wipe out safely.

Chapter 8: The rules. Why do surfers need rules? You'll find out in this chapter. (Hint: it has something to do with preventing surfing from being a contact sport.) You'll also learn the basic right-of-way rules and about localism and respect.

Chapter 9: Learning to turn. Once you can stand up on your board, the wave is your oyster; this chapter shows you how to ride your surfboard across the face of a wave, how wave shape affects what you can do on a wave, and ten easy steps to turning your board.

Chapter 10: The next level. Wondering where to go next after you've got the hang of catching waves, standing up, and turning? This chapter gives you a few options, including tackling bigger waves (with tips from *Blue Crush* surfer Kate Skarratt), surfing through winter, getting surf coaching, changing your surfboard (the pros and cons of longboards and shortboards), competitive surfing, and the joy of surf trips, including a few of North America's best surf destinations.

One last thing, before we set off: Throughout the book you'll see quotes from a few surfer girls at various stages of the learning process. If you want to know a bit more about them (and see what they look like), turn to Appendix 1: The surfer girls.

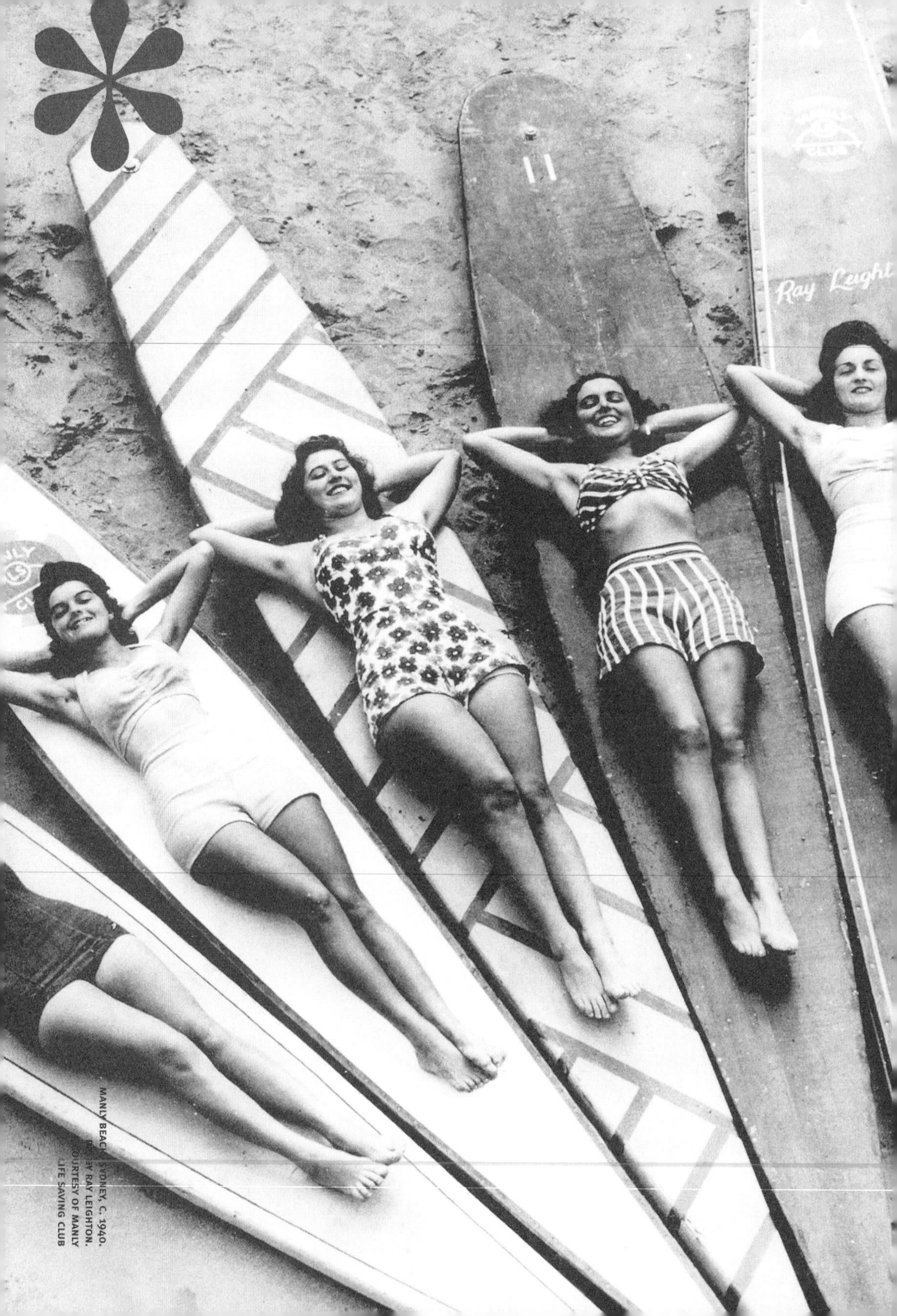

MANLY BEACH, SYDNEY, C. 1940.
PHOTO BY RAY LEIGHTON.
COURTESY OF MANLY
LIFE SAVING CLUB

CHAPTER **1**

looking
* back

In the beginning . . .

With more and more women now taking their place in surf spots around the world, gaining confidence and finding that they belong out there as much as anyone, it's tempting to think that women's surfing is a new phenomenon. But females have been surfing for longer than you think.

In fact you could say that women have always had a kinship with the waves. The ocean is, after all, female—ask any poet. Maybe it's because the sea can be so beautiful and full of life, stormy and quiet, gentle and powerful, all at once. There are myths about women surfing long ago in Tahiti, Aotearoa (New Zealand), and Rapa Nui (Easter Island). And don't tell the guys, but according to one Hawaiian legend, women even learned to surf before men: when Kamohoali'I, the shark god, taught Pele, the goddess of volcanoes, how to surf.

Why the history lesson?

Why is any of this important? It goes without saying that you need to look where you're going when you're learning something new, but a glance backward through time, learning about the people who cleared the path and understanding how surfing evolved, can be both informative and inspiring. If women could learn to surf—and surf well—when surfboards weighed a ton, there were no surf schools, and boardshorts and leashes were yet to be invented, then hey, maybe it's not so hard after all.

It's also important to know our roots. The history of surfing has been well documented over the years, but often with a subtle bias. You'd be hard pressed to find a surfer today who's never heard of Midget Farrelly, the first men's world surfing champion. But who's heard of Phyllis O'Donnell, the first women's world champion, who stood beside Midget on the winner's dais at the first World Championships, held at Sydney's Manly Beach in 1964?

It's not a conspiracy—just a side effect of the way events were recorded in those days and the amount of media coverage devoted to women's events—but it's not the full story either. Of course, a comprehensive history of surfing including the advances made by men and women would fill an entire book by itself. So the role of this chapter is to shine a light on a few of the women who have been part of the evolution of surfing. (By the way, if you're eager to get to the nitty-gritty of learning to surf, feel free to go straight to Chapter 2. That's the beauty of history: You can always come back to it later).

Think of it as looking back over your shoulder at all the dedicated surfer girls who have gone before you. Of course, women's surfing isn't separate from or superior to (or inferior to) men's surfing. But women are part of the bigger picture and, if the truth be known, always have been. In fact we're making history right now just by getting out there and making women's surfing visible once again.

Hawaii, A.D. 4

Imagine yourself in the middle of the Pacific Ocean, on a small group of islands that have always loomed large in surfing's history: Hawaii, the birthplace of modern surfing. Now turn back the clock two thousand years to A.D. 4 when Polynesians started coming ashore. It's hard to imagine a race of people more in sync with the ocean than the first Polynesians, particularly those who braved the long voyage to Hawaii. Of course, they already knew how to surf, but they did it lying down on short flat belly boards called *paipo*. It was the Hawaiians who took surfing up a notch, literally—by standing on longer surfboards.

Surfing was huge in Hawaii before European settlement, and it wasn't just a guy thing. Whole villages of men and women would surf together, sing songs to bring waves, and observe rituals and beliefs associated with the simple act of riding a wave. Surfing was even regarded as a kind of ocean-blessed foreplay; if a man and a woman rode a wave together, Hawaiian law permitted them to, er, get friendly on the sand when they got back to the beach.

Hawaiian social classes even extended past the shore break: There were surf breaks for royalty and surf breaks for commoners, and while Hawaiian princesses rode massive boards called *olo* that were up to 18 feet long (almost twice as long as the longest surfboards today), commoners rode shorter 12-foot boards called *alaia*. (The first surfboard to grace Australia's shores was actually an *alaia*. Manly Beach local C. D. Paterson lugged it back to Sydney from a trip to Hawaii in 1912. He tried to ride it but was so unsuccessful he gave it to his mom to use as an ironing board!)

1900–15: The first "beach girls"

This idyllic existence continued until 1778, when Captain James Cook made the first recorded European visit to the islands, bringing previously unheard-of diseases that decimated Hawaii's population from around half a million to barely forty thousand. In a few short years, Hawaii's surfers were almost wiped out. The ones who survived soon had to contend with the puritanical missionaries who arrived in 1820, dismissed surfing as un-Christian, and virtually outlawed wave-riding for everyone but the royal family.

Surfing languished in this forbidden zone for almost a hundred years until the early 1900s, when missionaries began to lose their grip on the islands. Unfortunately, new ways of life had been adopted in the meantime, which was bad news for Hawaiian women; instead of going surfing, they were now expected to spend all their time cooking, cleaning, and looking after the kids. For the first time in history, surfing had become "men only."

Eventually, however, the Hawaiians' longing for their favorite pastime won out. Hawaii became a holiday destination for visiting mainlanders during the early 1900s, and the local "beach boys" who hung out at Waikiki, the hub of the new tourism, started taking them out into the waves, first on outrigger canoes and then surfboards. This was a breath of fresh air for Hawaiian culture and resulted in many of Hawaii's women taking to the waves again. The newly formed Hui Nalu (Surf Club) even had two female members, **Mildred (Ladybird) Turner**, and Waikiki "beach girl" **Josephine (Jo) Pratt**, who became widely regarded as Hawaii's most accomplished female surfboard rider between 1909 and 1911.

1907: Surfing comes to the United States

Surfing officially graced the shores of mainland America in July 1907 when Hawaiian beach boy George Freeth started giving paid surfing demonstrations at Redondo Beach and Venice Beach, California. Although he wasn't the first person to surf in California— a handful of Hawaiian princes who were attending military school in California had demonstrated "surf sliding" in Santa Cruz as early as 1885—it was Freeth who really ignited surfing in America's consciousness.

Another Waikiki beach boy to attain surf-star status in the early 1900s was the gorgeously handsome champion swimmer Duke Kahanamoku. On his way to winning a gold medal for the 100-meter freestyle at the 1912 Olympics in Stockholm, Duke stopped in Southern California to give a few surfing demonstrations at Corona del Mar and Santa Monica and caused quite a stir among the SoCal locals. On his way back from Sweden, Duke also took the time to introduce surfing to the East Coast, surfing for the crowds in Atlantic City, New Jersey.

Duke also popularized tandem surfing—when two surfers

(usually a guy and a girl) ride the same board—which he demonstrated all over the world, including Sydney, Australia, in the summer of 1914–15.

1915: Surfing arrives in Australia

It's hard to imagine a more prehistoric era in the history of surfing than Australia in the early 1900s. Picture this: You're forbidden to swim during daylight hours (the ban on public bathing between 6 A.M. and 8 P.M. was lifted at Manly Beach in Sydney in 1902, and other beaches followed suit soon after); swimming zones are segregated for guys and girls; and when you do get in the water you have to wear a long-sleeved woolen swimsuit that's ten times heavier when it's wet than when it's dry.

Into this setting came the Duke, a bronzed Hawaiian swimming and surfing god, in 1915. Although initially invited by the New South Wales Swimming Association to give a public swimming demonstration, it was Duke's surfing skills that had the biggest impact on the Australian public. Australians had been surfing lying down on 4-to-5 foot wooden surfboards and body-surfing with wooden handboards—some had even heard about stand-up surfing in Hawaii and seen a couple of local surfers standing up—but stand-up surfing was still more of a rumor than a reality for most Aussie beachgoers at the time.

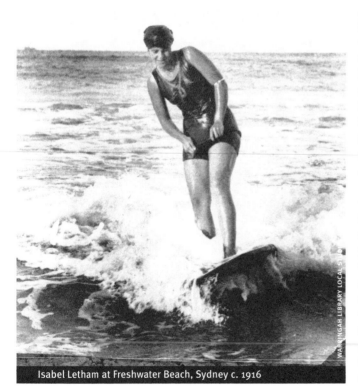

Isabel Letham at Freshwater Beach, Sydney c. 1916

It's something of a coup for women's surfing that one of the first Australians to stand up on a surfboard was a fifteen-year-old girl. **Isabel Letham** was just about to turn sweet sixteen when Duke made an appearance at Sydney's Freshwater Beach to give a demonstration of "Hawaiian-style surf-shooting." It was a rainy Sunday in January 1915, and several hundred Sydney-siders had turned out to watch Duke's unusual antics on the wave: first he paddled out lying down (instead of kneeling as most Aussies had done before then), and when he caught a wave he stood up and angled across it instead of heading straight toward the beach.

When Duke asked for a girl from the crowd to go tandem surfing with him, the organizers of the event knew just who to pick. Letham was renowned for her tomboyish behavior; at a time when most girls were embroidering hankies, she was spending every spare minute down at the beach swimming and bodysurf-

THE EVOLUTION OF THE HUMBLE BIKINI

It's probably safe to say that swimwear as we know it originated in ancient Rome, where murals have been found depicting women in two-piece bathing suits. But they were ahead of their time. Public swimming didn't take off among fair-skinned Europeans until the 1700s, and even then it was more "bathing"—that is, wading into the ocean—than actually swimming. That's why the first swimsuits were basically just dresses you could get wet; girls even sewed weights into the hems to stop their skirts from floating up and exposing their legs.

By 1900, most young women were pretty much over the whole Victorian self-denial thing and started spending more time in the water, although their swimsuits were still modest. Think knee-length wool dresses teamed with puffy pants called bloomers, long stockings, even special lace-up "swimming shoes." And they could be any color as long as it was black. Most girls also wore hats called bathing bonnets to keep the sun off the parts of their bodies that were exposed—a tan was thought to be so "working class."

By 1915, the year Isabel Letham first stood up on a surfboard and Californian women were beginning to discover the joys of surfing, swimming costumes began to get a bit more revealing. Some of them were even sleeveless! Things really started to heat up, however, in the 1930s and '40s when movie stars wore fitted feminine swimsuits, sometimes with jewelry and high heels. Cotton replaced wool as the fabric of choice and because it was lighter

when wet, it made swimming in the sea more than just a nice idea.

Then, in the summer of '46, French designer Louis Reard unveiled his skimpy two-piece creation at a Paris fashion show, saying it was so small "it revealed everything about the girl except her mother's maiden name." He originally called it "the Atome" but later decided on "the Bikini" because the United States had just begun testing nuclear bombs on Bikini Atoll in the Pacific. *Ooh la la*, the bikini as protest garment! Bikinis weren't popular right away, though—they were long regarded as suitable attire for strippers, not honest womenfolk, and were banned from the beaches of some Catholic countries.

By the 1950s, women started wanting to change their shapes, usually with cotton padding inside their tops, to suit the more revealing swimsuits, until the free-love seventies, when bra-burning spread to swimwear. Then came Lycra, with its "what you see is what you get" message.

Now we have the freedom to wear what we like when we go to the beach. So the next time you're dashing into the surf in your bikini and boardshorts, remember the pioneering girls who made life at the beach what it is today. As Hollywood's aquatic movie star Esther Williams, who virtually lived in her swimwear, once said, "A bathing suit is the least amount of clothing you're going to wear in public, so you better give it some thought." Hmm, that's worth thinking about.

ing. She was also a natural choice because Duke hadn't brought a surfboard with him to Australia and her dad had helped him to make a traditional Hawaiian surfboard from a log of sugar pine.

On the first few waves they paddled for, Letham was so scared, she made Duke stop because she said it felt like they were going over a cliff. Gentleman that he was, Duke did stop—the first few times—but he finally ignored her cries and took off on a wave, hauling her up by the scruff of her neck to stand beside him. They rode four waves that day, and by the time they returned to terra firma Letham was hooked. She became a dedicated surfer, teaching others to swim and surf in all conditions. In 1918 she traveled to America to find work as a Hollywood stuntwoman and was appointed Director of Swimming at the San Francisco Women's City Club, where she taught remedial swimming to disabled women. She was an inspiration to all women surfers right up until she died in 1995 at the age of ninety-five.

Soon everyone in Australia was surfing standing up. In fact surfing became so big that popular beaches such as Coolangatta on the Gold Coast introduced restricted surfing zones, punishable by board confiscation. Manly Council in Sydney even banned surfboards from the beach altogether until several board-aided rescues in 1923 forced it to reverse its decision.

1920s: The first surfer girls

Until the 1920s, surfing's popularity among women, outside Hawaii, was limited by one important factor: surfboards were *huge*. Think 12 feet long, made from solid timber, and weighing almost 100 pounds. Not only that but they didn't have any fins, which meant they were impossible to turn; if you did want to turn, you had to put one foot in the water (ever tried to keep your balance on a moving surfboard with one foot dragging in the sea?). At least it made surfing more sociable. Most surfers rode their boards straight to the beach, which meant that more than one surfer could ride each wave.

One way to get out there when surfboards were so cumbersome was to tag along with a guy. The first women surfers in Southern California often went tandem surfing with their boyfriends. They'd go to the beach together, ride the board together; then, if the girl was interested enough, she might take it up and get her own board. There were more independent-minded women, though, like the legendary **Mary Ann Hawkins**. In the tradition of Hawaiian surfers before her, Hawkins was an all-around waterwoman: surfer, bodysurfer, and long-distance swimmer. She was one of the first surfing females to earn the respect of the fledgling Californian surfing fraternity for her wave-riding throughout the 1930s and '40s and one of the first people to surf Palos Verdes, where she used to lug her 80-pound redwood surfboard up and down the cliffs on her way to and from the beach. For all this and more, Hawkins has been called the greatest woman surfer in the first half of the twentieth century.

Surfing got another boost during World War II when thousands of women (and men) were stationed at U.S. military bases in Hawaii. Some of them took up surfing; others just wrote home about the beautiful beaches and waves. This was the beginning of the annual winter pilgrimage of surfers to Hawaii for the big swells that hit the islands between December and March, a tradition that continues today; some of the most anticipated contests of the pro tour are those held in December at Sunset and Pipeline on the North Shore of Oahu, and on the island of Maui.

1950s: "Girl Boards"

In the late 1940s, using new materials developed during World War II, Californian shapers started making surfboards from a lightweight wood called balsa, which they'd salvaged from ex-navy life rafts. Balsa surfboards were a major breakthrough. Lighter and more buoyant, they made the waves accessible to more girls, not just muscle-bound guys.

In the 1950s, Californian shaper Joe Quigg made three balsa "Girl Boards" for three Malibu surfer girls: **Vicki Flaxman, Aggie Bane**, and **Robin Grigg**. Each girl painted her name and a design on her Girl Board, but what was really different about these surfboards was that they were curved from nose to tail, in contrast to the flat-as-a-plank boards of the time. As a result they were much easier to turn—they also allowed you to walk to the nose and do tricks—and when the guys saw how easily the girls were riding them, they all wanted one too.

Quigg went on to make surfboards for other surfer girls, one of whom was **Marge Calhoun**, who came to surfing through her work as a water stuntwoman in Hollywood. In 1958, Calhoun and fellow Californian **Eve Fletcher** (who had only learned to surf the year before, when she was thirty) flew to Hawaii to compete in the Makaha International contest—they paid legendary surfer Fred Van Dyke $100 to live in his panel truck for a month—and Calhoun subsequently won, on a 10-foot balsa board. There was no women's professional circuit back then, but this was the beginning of women competing in surfing.

1957–59: Gidget goes surfing

In 1957, surfing hit the mainstream thanks to a fifteen-year-old named **Kathy Kohner**, aka **Gidget**. After living in Europe for a year, Kohner and her family moved back to Malibu Beach, California. It was hot, it was summer, and Kohner hadn't made many new friends yet so her mom sent her down to the beach for some fresh air. She got more than that: Kohner started hanging out with the surfer boys who used to inhabit Malibu (literally: one guy called Tubesteak lived in a shack on the sand). The boys teased Kohner because not only was she the only girl hanging around, she was tiny—a mere 5'2" tall. Eventually one of them said to her, "You're a midget and a girl—you're a Gidget!"

Soon after that, Gidget bought herself a surfboard for $35 and taught herself how to surf by copying the guys. She was so fascinated by this new subculture, she started writing it all down in her diary and telling her family about it. Her dad, Hollywood screenwriter Frederick Kohner, saw the potential for a hit, and in 1957 wrote a novel called *Gidget: The Little Girl with Big Ideas*, which sold half a million copies and led to three Gidget movies (the first one was made in 1959), starring Sally Field and Sandra Dee; a 32-episode TV series; Gidget comics, games, and songs; as well as more than twenty beach-party movies throughout the sixties.

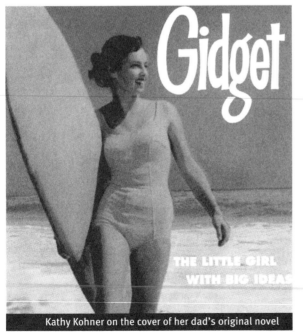
Kathy Kohner on the cover of her dad's original novel

Gidget Goes Hawaiian starred another Californian surfer, **Linda Benson**, who did all the surfing in the movie. Like Gidget, Benson learned to surf almost by chance. It was 1955, long before leashes were invented, and eleven-year-old Benson used to spend her free time down at Moonlight Beach in Southern California, wading into the water to retrieve lost boards after their riders wiped out. Then she started paddling the boards back out to the surfers. It wasn't long before one of them offered her a ride on his board; she stood up and caught a wave to the beach, and from that day on she was hooked. In 1959, at the age of fifteen, she entered and won the first U.S. Championships at Huntington Beach before heading to Hawaii to quench her thirst for bigger waves. Once there she became the first woman to surf Waimea Bay, the renowned big-wave spot on the North Shore. She was also one of the first surfers to "hang ten"—that is, walk to the nose of the board and hang all ten toes over the edge.

The 1960s: Surfing hits the big time

Surfing became huge in the late fifties and early sixties and, thanks to Gidget and her movies, women played an integral part. The Beach Boys' hit song "Surfer Girl" came out in 1963. Magazines such as *Life*, *Seventeen*, and *Sports Illustrated* started featuring stories and photos of surfers. Non-surfers even started using expressions like "hang ten" and "surf's up." There were beach parties, a surf-inspired dance called the "stomp," even surf fashion items like flower-print miniskirts: If you didn't surf back then, you wanted to look like you did.

It was also a time when surfers started going on surf trips up and down the coast—and farther afield—particularly after seeing Bruce Brown's classic 1966 surf flick, *The Endless Summer*, about a couple of surfers traveling the world in search of the perfect wave. *The Endless Summer* also brought international recognition to two surfer girls: Hawaiian **Bernie Ross** and Australian **Pearl Turton**.

Turton was already famous in Australia. In 1963, when surf contests were starting up all over the country, the sixteen-year-old from Sydney's northern beaches won the Women's Interstate Title (the equivalent of today's Australian Titles) held at Sydney's North Avalon. The contest was the biggest thing in Australian surfing at the time, and Turton, Australia's first women's surfing champion, became an overnight surf star: She appeared on the cover of the *Australian Women's Weekly*; she wrote the first-ever women's surfing column for *Surfabout* magazine, the first Australian surfing magazine; she even did live-to-air broadcasts on national TV wearing only her bikini.

The following year, 1964, the world got its first female surfing hero at the first World Championships, held at Manly Beach. It was one of the biggest surfing contests ever: more than 60,000 people crowded onto the popular Sydney beach for a glimpse of the latest surf stars in action. **Phyllis O'Donnell**, a surfer from the Tweed Coast in northern New South Wales and the 1964 Australian champion, blitzed the competition, including Linda Benson, who was tipped to win, and became the first women's world surfing champion.

HEY, WAXHEAD! If someone says this to you, take it as a compliment. It dates back to the sixties, when dedicated surfers used to carry their hefty surfboards on their heads, wax side down (wax is applied to the deck of a surfboard to keep you from slipping off when you're surfing). Avid surfers would get wax in their hair, hence the expression.

Joyce Hoffman was another competitive surfer who made her mark on the sixties. Although she came from a surfing family, it was her athleticism that led her to the waves. She excelled at many sports, including tennis, running, and skiing, and wanted to be the best in the world at something, but it wasn't until Hoffman's family moved to California's Capistrano Beach that she fell in love with surfing, which ironically had limited prospects for women back then. But her competitive drive found expression, and she was soon winning every contest she entered. She went on to earn five world titles between 1966 and 1971 and was the first woman to surf the legendary Pipeline (so-called because when it breaks over the shallow coral reef, it forms a hollow "pipe") on Hawaii's North Shore.

From longboards to shortboards

In 1960, foam-core surfboards (like today's surfboards) replaced the old wooden boards. This was a major innovation in design for two reasons: foam is much lighter than timber, and it is easier to cut into shape. The sixties were all about experimentation, so it wasn't long before surfers started chopping a foot or two off the nose of their boards, just to see how they'd go. They soon found out: Shorter surfboards were much easier to turn than the old 9-foot longboards, which meant you could do more on a wave.

With the transition from longboards to lighter and more maneuverable shortboards, a whole new generation of female surfers started showing the world what they could do. Two of the most prominent were **Margo Oberg** (née Godfrey) and **Lynne Boyer**, who played a long-running game of cat-and-mouse and won five world titles between them, from 1977 to 1981.

California's Margo Oberg started competing on longboards in 1964, and by the time she was thirteen she was ranked fourth in the world. Then, just before the 1968 world championships, she switched to a shortboard—which she loved because of her small build—and won at the age of fifteen (what is it about these fifteen-year-old surfer girls?). She went on to win three more world titles in 1977, 1980, and 1981, and was one of the most phenomenal surfers of all time, not least because she had the longest pro-surfing career of any female before or since: She competed for more than thirty years.

Lynne Boyer, by contrast, grew up on the East Coast, surfing on rubber mats and Styrofoam boards near her family's summer house in Wildwood, New Jersey, before her family moved to Hawaii in

1968, when she was eleven. Before long she began competing and became Oberg's chief rival, winning two world titles, in 1978 and 1979. Boyer dropped out of competitive surfing in 1984 to pursue her passion for painting and is now an acclaimed artist; she returned to competitive surfing in 1997, a mellower but no less talented version of her former self.

Joyce Hoffman neatly sums up the influence she and other Californian female surfers had on women's surfing of the time: "Marge Calhoun and her daughters really made surfing look possible for women and showed them that it was more than a sport. It's a mind-set, a lifestyle. Linda Benson pushed the sport. She was the first one to try to do it like the boys, with a more aggressive style. Then I took it and tried to do it exactly like the guys at that time. Margo Oberg came along and took it to the next level and opened the sport up to a lot of women through the longevity of her career. There have been other influential women along the way, but I think we set the pace and set the sport in motion. . . . That's just the luck of when we were born." (From p. 53 of *Girl in the Curl* by Andrea Gabbard, Seal Press, 2000)

Meanwhile, back in Australia, Victorian **Gail Couper** came to be regarded as one of the best Aussie female surfers of the sixties and seventies: she won the contest at Bells Beach (now the longest-running surfing contest in the world) nine times, she won the Australian titles five times, and she received fourteen Victorian titles. "There were quite a lot of other women into surfing," Couper told *SurfGirl* magazine in 2001. "We had a board club in Lorne with about ten women, and there were lots of other clubs along the coast who we'd compete against. . . . It felt like we were pioneering things."

The 1970s: The Dark Ages

Surfing became more high performance throughout the late seventies and eighties—particularly after the introduction in 1981 of the provocatively named Thruster, a three-fin board designed by Sydney surfer Simon Anderson—and the gap between men's and women's surfing widened into a chasm. Anti-female comments such as "No chicks on sticks!" and "No boobs in tubes!" were directed at any girl brave enough to paddle out. Some male surfers even claimed that women were too "top heavy" to balance on a surfboard. Those women who managed to prove the guys wrong, such as Margo Oberg and Lynne Boyer, were dismissed as freaks and regarded as unfeminine. So much for "free love"!

Surfing also became more competitive. Power and speed were valued over grace and style, and professional surfing as we know it began. In 1976, a women's pro tour was developed by the newly formed organization that ran the men's surfing tour, the International Professional Surfing (IPS).

THE PROBLEM WITH PRO SURFING

Women's pro contests were originally held alongside the men's, but there were problems with this format. Because of the dominance of male surfing, it was not unusual for the men's heats to be held in the best surf, relegating women to lesser-quality waves; lack of sponsorship meant that female pro surfers won much less prize money than the male pros; and media coverage at events focused on the male competitors.

So, in 1979, a group of female pro surfers including Margo Oberg, Lynne Boyer, and Rell Sunn, led by 1976 world champion Jericho Poppler, set up their own professional organization, **Women's Professional Surfing (WPS).** Their mission: to increase sponsorship and media coverage of women's surfing. There had been localized movements before this: In 1975, Poppler and Mary Setterholm set up the **Women's International Surfing Association (WISA),** which sponsored and organized women's pro-am surfing events along the California coast for seventeen years (the last WISA contest was held in 1991). And the **Australian Women's Surfriders Association (AWSA)** was formed in 1978 with Isabel Letham, then seventy-eight, as patron.

While all these organizations had their successes, the situation didn't change dramatically, so when the Association of Surfing Professionals (ASP) was established in 1982 to run the world tour, the women gladly joined, hoping that being part of one large organization would give them more negotiating power. But again, the status of women's surfing didn't improve. As Layne Beachley put it at the time, "Currently, we're competing with the guys for a five-day contest period. We're always put in the water either at the end of the day when no one's around or when it turns onshore or when it's low tide and crappy. We just seem to be treated as a sideshow to the men's tour."

Finally, in April 2000, five of the world's best women surfers—Rochelle Ballard, Layne Beachley, Megan Abubo, Kate Skarratt, and Prue Jeffries—took matters into their own hands by creating **International Women's Surfing (IWS).** Their main aim was to increase the value of the women's pro tour, specifically by creating a series of women-only events that could secure their own sponsorship dollars and media coverage.

So far, so good. In 2004, five of the women's seven World Championship Tour events were women only. According to Rochelle Ballard, women's surfing has come a long way in four years: "The IWS has definitely been a key element in progressing the future of women's surfing. We're now recognized by the media as the elite of our sport and not a sideshow to the men." There's still room for improvement, of course—the prize money for the 2004 women's tour came to only $448,300 (the total men's prize money in 2004 was $2.86 million)—but, as Ballard points out, the IWS is about more than improving the lot of pro surfers. "The IWS is also involved at the grassroots of the sport, helping kids develop their talents with surf camps and a new series of one-star contests in America. It's basically surfers using our resources to give something back and create opportunities for the next generation."

The 1980s: Surfing gets serious

Women's surfing really started taking itself seriously in the 1980s. In 1984, **Frieda Zamba** from Daytona Beach, Florida, began her four-world-title reign, bringing her natural athleticism to surfing and giving new meaning to the term "performance surfing." Zamba was the first world champion to come from Florida, a place renowned for fickle waves, but she wasn't the last. Four-time world champ Lisa Andersen and six-time men's champion Kelly Slater are both from Florida.

One of the most interesting trends in women's surfing since the pro tour began in 1976 is the tug-of-war between America and Australia in the quest for world titles. Although the pro tour has always been, and continues to be, a multinational affair, American surfers initially dominated women's surfing in a big way, winning every world title from 1976 until 1987, when **Wendy Botha**, who honed her skills in South Africa's chilly shark-infested waves, won her first world title. (Botha later became an Australian citizen and won three more world titles in 1989, 1991, and 1992.)

Then came **Pam Burridge** from Sydney's Manly Beach. Even before she became Australia's first pro surfer in 1982, Burridge's powerful surfing attracted considerable attention; she was even dubbed "the new Margo Oberg." Once she was on the tour, however, the pressure intensified. The Australian media wanted to see an Australian win the world title, and Burridge seemed the perfect candidate to carry their dreams. Finally, after being the "bridesmaid" four years in a row and struggling under the weight of so many expectations, she realized the dream of every Aussie surfer girl: In 1990, at the age of twenty-five, Pam Burridge was crowned world champion. (Burridge competed for another nine years after her win and then retired to the New South Wales south coast; she named her first child after Isabel Letham, her surfing mentor.)

Australia gained another champion in 1993 when Bondi surfer **Pauline Menczer** won the world title despite often-crippling back pain. Menczer has gone on to become a much-loved veteran of the tour, still competing after more than sixteen years. Another Aussie surfer who made an impact in the nineties was **Jodie Cooper**, from Albany in Western Australia. Although she never won a world title, Cooper earned respect for her gutsy power-surfing in big waves—and her stylish moves in *Point Break* (she was the stunt surfer for Keanu Reeves's surfer girlfriend, played by Lori Petty).

BOARDS FOR YOUR BOOBS

In the early 1990s, a group of surfer girls in Byron Bay in northern NSW, Australia, received a government grant to design a surfboard specifically for women. The resulting "boob board" had depressions in the deck for those, er, delicate parts of the female anatomy. But their moment in the sun was brief: Apparently the boards were too difficult to make in a DD cup. Believe it or not. . . .

The Lisa and Layne show

Australia's winning streak continued until 1994, when Florida-born **Lisa Andersen** took center stage. When Andersen ran away from home at the age of sixteen to escape her warring parents, she left them a note: "I'm leaving to become the world champion of women's surfing." Ten years later, in 1994, she won the first of four consecutive world titles—the first time any female surfer had ever achieved that feat. One of the most stylish surfers ever, Andersen brought grace back to surfing, at a time when it was dominated by power surfers, and became one of the first pro surfers to achieve rock-star status in the surfing world. In 1995 she even became the first woman to grace the cover of *Surfer* magazine with the cover line: "Lisa Andersen surfs better than you."

Persistent back problems forced Andersen to withdraw temporarily from competitive surfing in 1998, the year **Layne Beachley**, originally from Sydney's Manly Beach, won her first world title. And in case anyone dared to suggest that Andersen's absence helped Beachley win, Layne won the world title again in 1999 and then in 2000 (when Andersen returned to the tour) and followed through with wins in 2001, 2002, and 2003.

Beachley has now won six consecutive world titles, a feat never before achieved by any other surfer, male or female, in the history of surfing. It's no wonder she has been called "the greatest all-round female surfer of all time"; not only does she excel in the competitive arena and in small waves, but she pushes the limits of what women were thought to be capable of in big surf too. She pioneered tow-in surfing for women in the nineties, when she started spending large parts of her year living at Sunset Beach on Hawaii's North Shore with her then partner, big-wave legend Ken Bradshaw.

While women surfers have long been charging Hawaii's big waves, they're now tackling even bigger ones—waves that are so big they can only be caught by being towed into them with the aid of a Jet Ski. In January 2001, Beachley caught the biggest wave a woman has ever ridden, when she was towed into a 55-foot monster at Outer Log Cabins, a reef about a mile off the coast of Hawaii's North Shore.

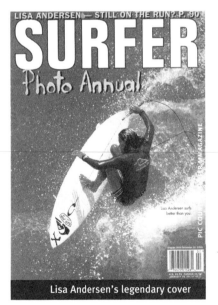

Lisa Andersen's legendary cover

The rise and rise of women's surfing

Women's surfing really started booming with the "girl power" vibe of the 1990s. In 1991 Quiksilver created Roxy, the world's first girls' surf brand, a move which all other major brands have since followed. In 1994 former pro surfer Debbie Beacham and Donna Olson co-produced *Surfer Girl,* the first women's surfing movie, a 16-mm documentary that featured five former pro surfers—Debbie Beacham, four-time world champions Frieda Zamba and Wendy Botha, Jodie Cooper, and 1990 world champion Pam Burridge—riding perfect waves and reflecting on the surfing life while on a surf trip in Tavarua, Fiji. In 1995, *Wahine,* the first women's surfing magazine, was launched in California by Marilyn Edwards and journalist Elizabeth Glazner, who first met in 1993, when Edwards was returning to surfing after a long break and Glazner was

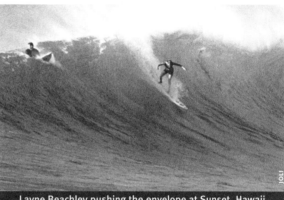

Layne Beachley pushing the envelope at Sunset, Hawaii

BIG WAVE BRAVADO

Women have always been riding big waves—surfing originated, after all, in Hawaii, the epicenter of big-wave surfing—but in recent years they seem to be tackling bigger and meaner ones. Santa Cruz surfer **Sarah Gerhardt** is a case in point. One winter's day in February 1999, after honing her big-wave skills in Hawaii, Gerhardt took off on a 25-foot monster and became the first woman ever to surf Mavericks, a treacherous break half a mile off the coast of Half Moon Bay in Northern California, renowned for its achingly cold water, big sharks, and long hold-downs. Since then she's been a regular at the annual invitation-only Quiksilver/Men Who Ride Mountains event held there—and organizers are wondering if they'll need to change the name of the contest if she wins.

Gerhardt is just one of a new breed of big-wave chargers. **Rochelle Ballard** and **Megan Abubo** became the first all-girl tow-in surfing team when they did the stunt surfing for *Blue Crush* in Hawaii in 2002. And when Australian surfer **Kate Skarratt** surfed the usually crowded Pipeline virtually by herself for a scene in the movie, she called it "a milestone for women's surfing."

Meanwhile, back on the mainland, another Santa Cruz surfer, **Jamilah Star,** is getting a reputation as a big-wave surfer to watch. In the winter of 2003–4, Star not only became the second woman in history to surf Mavericks, she also paddled into a 50-foot wave at Waimea Bay on Hawaii's North Shore, which earned her the cover of *Surf Life for Women*'s spring 2004 issue. Star is now in training for tow-in surfing at another California big-wave break, the Cortes Bank, 100 miles off the coast of San Diego.

learning to surf. Water Girl, the first all-girl surf shop, opened in Encinitas, California, in 1995 too. And in 1996 Isabelle (Izzy) Tihanyi set up Surf Diva, the world's first surf school for women and girls, based in La Jolla, California.

In the summer of 2002, the world fell in love with surfer girls all over again when *Blue Crush*, a Hollywood movie about three girl surfers living on the North Shore of Hawaii, was released. It was the first of its kind: a feature film that portrayed the surfing lifestyle with credibility. It also showed the world some of the most talented female surfers on the planet: pro surfers Rochelle Ballard, Megan Abubo, Keala Kennelly, and Kate Skarratt. Not only were they able to keep their bikinis on in the powerful waves, a feat in itself, but Skarratt in particular surfed Pipeline like no other woman before her. *Blue Crush* also showed women competing in the Pipe Masters—a pipe dream for future pro surfers (in real life the contest has always excluded women).

Now more and more girls are learning to surf, experiencing their own "'blue crush" on the ocean and the surfing lifestyle. Competitively, women such as Peru's **Sofia Mulanovich** and Australian **Chelsea Georgeson** are surfing more radically than ever before, while surf breaks all over the world are witnessing a golden age in women's surfing. Ten percent of Australia's estimated 2.3 million surfers are female (Source: Surfing Australia). That figure is even higher in the United States, where women's surfing is the fastest growing sport in the country: 37 percent of America's 2.1 million surfers are female, up from 19 percent just two years ago, according to Board Trac market research (2003).

Surfer girls now have their own surf shops, surf videos, surf magazines, boardshorts, wetsuit brands, and surf contests. There are female surfing instructors who teach at all-girl surf schools, female surfboard shapers, and women's surf camps. Best of all, it's no longer unusual to see another girl out in the water, and in some places girl surfers even outnumber the guys. Women's surfing has truly come into its own. Go, girls!

KNOW YOUR WORLD CHAMPIONS

 Women's champions since pro surfing began

1976 Jericho Poppler (USA)	1990 Pam Burridge (Australia)
1977 Margo Oberg (Hawaii)	1991 Wendy Botha (Australia)
1978 Lynne Boyer (Hawaii)	1992 Wendy Botha (Australia)
1979 Lynne Boyer (Hawaii)	1993 Pauline Menczer (Australia)
1980 Margo Oberg (Hawaii)	1994 Lisa Andersen (USA)
1981 Margo Oberg (Hawaii)	1995 Lisa Andersen (USA)
1982 Debbie Beacham (USA)	1996 Lisa Andersen (USA)
1983 Kim Mearig (USA)	1997 Lisa Andersen (USA)
1984 Frieda Zamba (USA)	1998 Layne Beachley (Australia)
1985 Frieda Zamba (USA)	1999 Layne Beachley (Australia)
1986 Frieda Zamba (USA)	2000 Layne Beachley (Australia)
1987 Wendy Botha (South Africa)	2001 Layne Beachley (Australia)
1988 Frieda Zamba (USA)	2002 Layne Beachley (Australia)
1989 Wendy Botha (Australia*)	2003 Layne Beachley (Australia)

*Wendy Botha became an Australian citizen in 1989.

The story so far ...

A timeline of women's surfing

Isabel Letham becomes the first Australian woman to stand up on a surfboard when she surfs with Hawaiian Duke Kahanamoku. **1915**

1950 After World War II, surfboard shapers start making lighter balsa-wood surfboards, opening up surfing to women.

Gidget, the movie, brings surfing—and surfer girls—into mainstream culture. Linda Benson wins the first U.S. championships at Huntington Beach, California. **1959**

1964 Aussie Phyllis O'Donnell becomes the world's first women's surfing champion.

Joyce Hoffman wins the first of five world titles. **1966**

1968 Margo Oberg wins the first of four world titles at age fifteen.

The first women's pro surfing circuit is introduced. **1976**

1978 Lynne Boyer wins the first of two world titles.

Women's Pro Surfing (WPS) is formed by Jericho Poppler and other pro surfers. **1979**

1982 Pam Burridge becomes Australia's first female professional surfer.

Frieda Zamba from Florida wins her first of four world titles. **1984**

1987 South African (later Australian) Wendy Botha wins the first of four world titles.

Pam Burridge wins the world title. Hawaiian Rochelle Ballard turns pro. **1990**

Lisa Andersen from Florida wins the first of four consecutive world titles. **1993**

1994 Aussie Pauline Menczer wins the world title.

1995 *Wahine,* the world's first women's surfing magazine, is launched in the US. Water Girl, the first women's surf shop, opens in California.

Lisa Andersen graces the cover of *Surfer* magazine. Surf Diva surf school is set up in La Jolla, California. **1996**

1998 Layne Beachley wins her first world title. Hawaiian soul surfer, Rell Sunn, dies after a long struggle with cancer.

Blue Crush, the first Hollywood movie about women surfers, creates a "surfer girl" boom. **2002**

2003 Layne Beachley achieves a first in the history of surfing: six consecutive world titles.

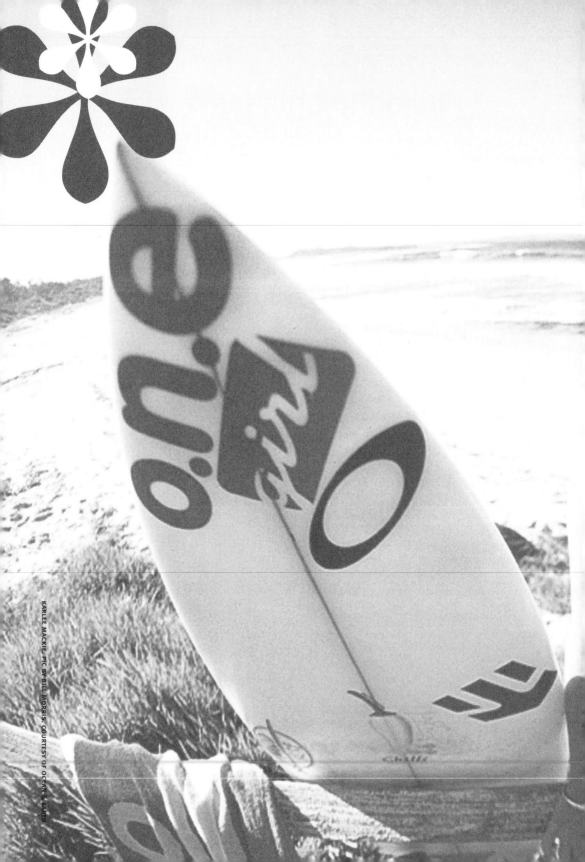

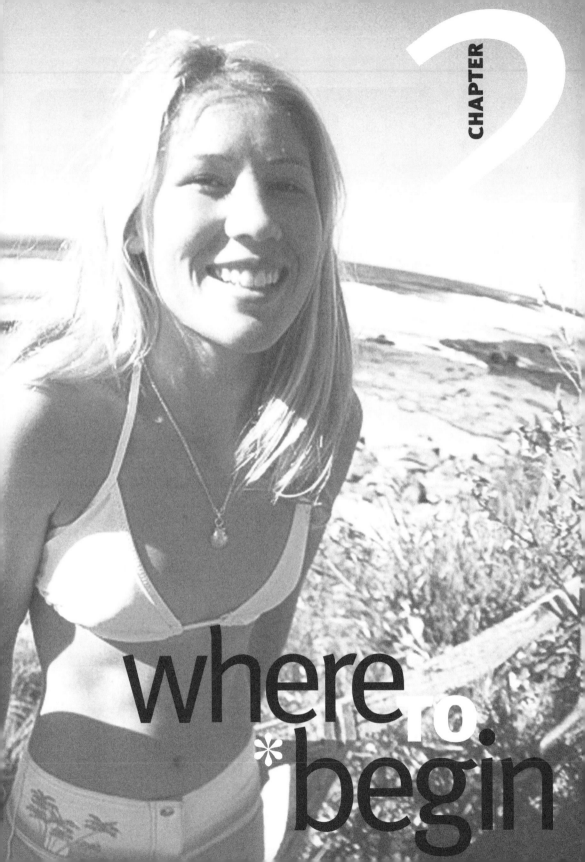

where *to. begin

Learn:

What's so great about surfing. **What skills you need to learn to surf.** How bodysurfing, bodyboarding, skateboarding, and snowboarding can help your surfing. **What surf schools can and can't teach you and the pros and cons of surf lessons.** How dangerous is surfing, really? **How surfing changes your body.**

✳

Start where you are . . .

So here you are, standing on the precipice of being a surfer. It's a good idea before you actually *do* anything to just check where you are. Where are you starting from? Have you spent much time in the ocean? Have you ever been on a surfboard, bodyboard, skateboard, or snowboard? How well can you swim? These are all factors worth thinking about, but the most important thing is to start where *you* are, not where you think you should be or where other surfers might have started.

The journey of a thousand miles really does start with one step. There's not a surfer out there today who didn't go through the dorky beginner phase, when they didn't know their wax comb from their nose guard. Even the hottest surfer at your local break was once a kook (that's surf slang for beginner).

One more thing before we set off: considering all the time and effort you're going to be putting in to learning the art of surfing, it's worth asking yourself why you want to do it. People surf for all sorts of reasons. For fun and fitness, to do something social with their friends, to get some time out from a busy life, to be in the ocean or in nature, or for all of the above. Why do *you* want to do it? Whatever your answer, it'll give you an idea of how much time you'll want to put in—and what you can expect to achieve.

Having said that, it's important from the start not to set your expectations too high or to have too rigid an idea of where you want to end up, particularly if you've never tried surfing before. You might decide that bodyboarding's more your style, or you might find that you want to compete in surf comps or try a longboard or a kneeboard; the possibilities are endless. So go easy on yourself. See how you feel at each step of the way, and know that you can adjust your goals at any time.

What's so great about surfing?

In a nutshell: lots of things! Everyone develops her own relationship to surfing, and when you start surfing you'll find your own reasons to love it. But for now, allow me to share a few of the things that have kept me surfing for more than a decade.

What I love about surfing is the thrill factor. When you're traveling along a wave, it's just the most incredibly buzzy feeling. I can't describe it. It actually gives you energy. You can come running out after a really good session and drive everyone bananas raving about it. And when you keep trying and it all comes together, it feels like such an achievement.

*10 things I love about surfing

1 It's fun, pure and simple, with no artificial colors or flavors. There's no better feeling than riding along the face of a wave and then paddling back out with a huge grin on your face.

2 It keeps you in touch with the natural world, which adds another dimension to an otherwise city-bound life. Go for a surf and you can't help but notice which way the wind's blowing, if it's low or high tide, and whether there are fish or sea birds around this time of year. Being a surfer makes you more weather-conscious, too, because you want to be able to predict swells and be ready for them.

3 It's simple. Think about it: all you need, really, is a surfboard and a few waves. Not only that, but the waves are free!

4 The sense of community. Yes, surfing is a great way to meet guys—the odds are in your favor, and you know you'll have at least one thing in common. But I also love the way you can fall into conversation with another surfer and find out about the new swell working its way up the coast, the good waves at a nearby beach, or the whale that was sighted yesterday. Without any planning whatsoever, you'll meet up with people you know out in the water, simply by virtue of the fact that you've all converged on the best spot to surf that day.

6 It's good all-over exercise. Surfing sculpts your body, toning your upper arms, shoulders, stomach, and legs like almost nothing else— and without you even realizing it!

5 It teaches you patience, whether you're waiting for that elusive last wave before you head in, waiting for the next set, or waiting for the flat spell to end so you can go surfing again. Surfers talk a lot about searching for waves, but we often overlook surfing's quieter sister: patience. In a world that values control, it's nice to know you can't hurry the ocean.

7 It's peaceful. Some city beaches can be aggravating, but even in the city you can often find a peak or a whole beach to yourself. At those times, surfing soothes the soul, giving you breathing space in your life and a chance to stop and just *be* (until your next wave). It helps you get things on land back in perspective too.

8 It builds your confidence, and that spreads to all areas of your life. If I can surf, what else can I do? Not only that, but it gives you stories to tell—about that amazing last wave you got yesterday, or your last surf trip up the coast, or the wipeout that all your friends teased you about for a week.

9 It's humbling. You might feel ten feet tall after riding your first wave all the way to the beach, but you can also get the whipping of your life if you're not paying attention. Surfing gives you an appreciation of the ocean's power and lets you see it in all its moods. You can never dominate the ocean; the best you can hope for is to be able to play in it.

10 It's beautiful. Summer sunsets when the ocean is as smooth as glass and the sky's colors set the sea on fire. Gloomy steel-colored days when raindrops splash into the water around you like diamonds. Full-circle rainbows in the spray off the back of a wave. Another surfer crouched inside the eye of a perfect barrel. The show never stops.

ANNA: Today we had a huge pod of dolphins swimming around us and playing, with two babies so close you could touch them. They were swimming under our boards, riding the waves; it was just awesome being out there with them. And so sunny and warm as well—the water was about 75 degrees; we were all surfing in bikinis.

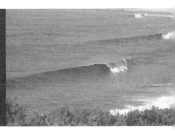

What skills do you need?

There are people who have never surfed before who just grab a friend's surfboard, paddle out, and start surfing. They're what's known, in common surfing parlance, as *freaks*. Most of us learn the hard way: by learning skills, practicing them, trying and practicing some more, and improving in small stages that feel like giant leaps, until we eventually feel competent enough to call ourselves surfers.

But there are ways to prepare yourself, mentally and physically, for the arduous (but fun!) task ahead.

How fit should you be?

There's no easy way to say this: learning to surf can be hard work. Your body isn't going to be "'surfing fit." Your shoulders and back will ache from paddling. You won't know the shortcuts that experienced surfers take to minimize effort, such as using rips to paddle out. You're going to be spending quite a bit of time in the whitewater, which can be physically draining because it tosses you around. Plus, you've got a big board to hold on to and wrestle with.

Now for the good news. While it's true that the best way to train for surfing is actually to go surfing, there are other ways to prepare yourself. As with any activity, the fitter you are, the more you're going to enjoy it—and that is, after all, what it's all about. A good level of fitness and stamina will help you to stay out in the water longer without getting tired, catch more waves because you'll have more energy, and handle wipeouts more easily without panicking.

You're going to need some upper-body fitness—particularly in your triceps, the muscles at the back of your upper arms. Swimming laps, preferably in salt water or, even better, in the ocean, is a great way to get yourself ready for all the paddling you're going to be doing. It will also help your aerobic fitness, which will help your general stamina and endurance—so you can surf longer and fast-track the learning process—as will anything else that gives you a cardiovascular workout such as cycling or running. You can also use light weights and do push-ups for upper body fitness.

Your legs need to have some strength too, because that gives you the stability—and, later, the power to turn—that you need when you're standing on your surfboard. Try soft sand running, squats, or stair running, or swim a few laps with a kickboard and flippers.

✳tip

Don't let lack of fitness become an excuse to put off learning to surf. Remember: start where you are. If you're not as trim, taut, and terrific as you'd like to be, don't worry; surfing will soon work its magic on your fitness levels.

If your back's strong, you'll be able to paddle strongly—try lying on your stomach and lifting your chest off the ground, making sure not to strain your neck. That'll help to strengthen those large muscles along your spine, which will help you to paddle your board without your back getting so tired.

Can you swim?

This might seem like a stupid question, but you'd be surprised how many people, particularly those who haven't spent much time near the ocean, learn to surf without being able to swim very well (or at all). If you can't swim, learn before you surf. If you're not a strong swimmer, do some laps to get yourself stronger before you start surfing. You don't have to be an Olympic athlete, but you should be able to swim at least 100 yards or two laps of an Olympic-size swimming pool and feel reasonably comfortable in the ocean. If you live near the beach, try doing swim training in the sea (preferably where there are no waves). Being a competent swimmer will give you a lot more confidence in the water. It'll also make paddling easier—and paddling is a big part of being a good surfer: Not only does it get you out there, it allows you to catch more waves and paddle back out easily after each ride.

Being a strong swimmer is also a safety issue. Sure, your board will keep you afloat in an emergency—but what happens if you lose your board and have to swim to the beach? If you're a good swimmer and have enough energy, it's no big deal. If not, you're not only endangering yourself, you're risking the safety of those who might try to rescue you. One of my friends once rescued a Japanese surfer who lost his board and was in danger of drowning. When they eventually dragged themselves onto the beach, over rocks that cut both of them to ribbons and dinged my friend's board, the guy confessed that he'd never learned to swim!

Have you ever been in the surf?

This might seem like another obvious question, particularly if you've lived on the coast all your life. But even if you've never seen a wave, you can still learn to surf, because once you start getting out in the water on a regular basis, you'll find that surfing teaches you more about the ocean than almost anything else.

Wave knowledge is not something you can learn from a book. It's gained from spending quality time with our mother the ocean. The way the ocean behaves can differ from country to country or from coast to coast, so it's important to look, listen, and learn about the place where you're going to be spending most of your learn-to-surf time. And the more time you spend in and around the

*tip

You should always be able to swim to the beach from where you're surfing. So don't sit out too far if you're not a strong swimmer. Be aware of how tired you are throughout your surf and keep a safety margin, a reserve of energy in case you can't get a wave in and have to paddle or swim back to the beach.

ocean, the more you'll realize how much there is to know. Things like how to dive under whitewater, how to keep your balance when you're walking out through the surf and waves are breaking around you, and never turning your back on the ocean (when you're in the water or at the water's edge—you're pretty safe when you're in the parking lot!).

You can give yourself a head start by:

- Swimming in the surf. Practice ducking under the whitewater; open your eyes underwater and look at how deep the whitewater of the breaking wave goes.
- Snorkeling or swimming with goggles at your local beach. Is there sand on the bottom? Are there any rocks? Does the bottom slope evenly up to the beach or are there holes and mounds of sand all over the place?
- Sitting quietly on the beach or on a rock overlooking the sea and studying the ocean. Watch how the waves form, where and how they break, whether there are any currents moving along the beach or back out to sea.

Ever been bodysurfing or bodyboarding?

If you grew up anywhere near a beach, chances are you already have quite a bit of wave knowledge. If, however, you haven't been in the ocean much, bodysurfing and bodyboarding (aka boogieboarding, after the first bodyboard, the Morey Boogie) are two great ways to get firsthand experience of waves before you get onto a surfboard. Best of all, both can be done in the safest area on the beach: usually between the swimming flags under the watchful gaze of the lifeguards.

The best thing about **bodysurfing** is that you don't need any equipment (other than a bikini that won't come off at the first hint of whitewater), and you can do it anywhere there are breaking waves. A good way to start bodysurfing is just to wade into the water as far as you feel comfortable. Before you even try to catch a wave, get used to the sensation of the waves hitting you; feel how much force there is in them, practice staying on your feet instead of getting knocked over; and practice facing the oncoming waves and diving or bobbing down under them.

Bodysurfing is as easy as standing in waist-deep water and throwing yourself in front of some whitewater by pushing off from the sand with your feet. When you get a bit more confident, you can try catching breaking (green) waves. This requires a bit more experience, since you have to launch yourself into the wave at the right time. Too early, and the wave will break on top of you; too

KAITLYN:
Boogieboarding's cool—it helped me to understand the ocean and how it works and it got me comfortable in bigger waves, which helped me make the transition to a surfboard. One time I was talking to a girl out in the water, and she said she started boogieboarding and picked up surfing really easily, so that made me think I should try it. That's how I started surfing.

late, and the wave will pass you by. Flippers are a good idea if you're going to go out of your depth and you want to catch unbroken waves—the trick with catching waves is to match the speed of the wave, and flippers help greatly in this. When you're "surfing," keep your arms either by your sides or out in front of you and look where you're going. (This is also important if it's crowded, to avoid plowing headfirst into one of your fellow swimmers.)

Bodyboarding is another great way to get surf experience. You can actually ride waves as you would on a surfboard, but you don't have to think about standing up, and the fun starts as soon as you catch your first wave! You'll need a bodyboard, a leash (to attach the board to your wrist) and a pair of flippers (also called fins).

As with bodysurfing, start in the whitewater, or foam, where there's no chance of being dumped and you can ride all the way to the sand. Carry your board out and start where you can still stand; then you won't have to tire yourself out by having to kick and paddle. Practice lying on your board. The back edge of the bodyboard should be where your legs meet your torso, so your whole body (except for your legs) is resting on it.

When you're ready, turn your board to the beach and throw yourself in front of some whitewater. Try to keep your legs together (it's more streamlined) and hang on to the front edge of your bodyboard with both hands, or put one hand there and the other on one side (this will help you to lean into the face of the wave and turn later on). When you progress to deeper water, you'll have to kick more to get onto waves—this is when a pair of flippers comes in handy.

How about skateboarding or snowboarding?

Surfers have always been into skateboarding and, more recently, snowboarding, the idea being that when you're skating or boarding you're standing sideways on a board (as in surfing) and moving down a sloping surface. But are they really so similar?

There's no doubt that skating and snowboarding can give you a feel for the way you can move on a surfboard. If you skate or snowboard you'll probably have good balance and a certain amount of core strength in your legs and torso, and when you get to the part where you have to turn your surfboard, you'll be streets ahead of anyone who doesn't have any experience with board sports. The things they don't teach you are how to get to your feet on a moving surface, how to catch a wave, and all about the weather and the way waves behave.

DEBORAH: Snowboarding really helps you with balance, to know where your center is, and with that feeling of fearlessness—you're facing down the mountain and making that leap of faith that you're going to turn on your edge. I feel like that with surfing too; you have to get it out of your head and put it in your body.

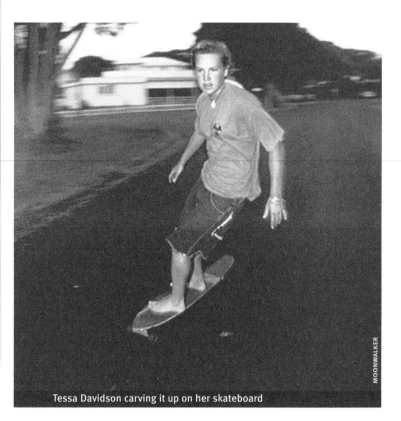

Tessa Davidson carving it up on her skateboard

Skateboarding is also a great way to practice surf moves when there are no waves or you can't get to the beach—you can keep trying the same move over and over until you get it—while snowboarding, particularly in powder, gives you a feel for how to carve turns on a surfboard.

But I'm not like all the other girls (or guys) who surf!

It's normal to feel out of place when you're learning something new. Everyone else doing it looks like they've got it all together; they look so cool, and they can do everything you can't (yet). They might dress differently from you or listen to different music or talk differently. When I learned to surf there were no other girls surfing, and I felt like an alien compared to the guys who surfed at my local beach; I was in my twenties, drove a hatchback, and didn't especially like death metal music. But the more I just got out there and tried to surf, the more I realized that there are many different kinds of people who surf, and all you can do is be the kind of surfer you are. Bring diversity to the lineup! Wear what you want to wear, not what you think you should wear. Listen to the kind of music that gets you grooving. Basically, just bring yourself to surfing; you don't have to become a clone of anyone else.

Should you have lessons?

Now that you've prepared yourself as much as is humanly possible without actually getting wet, it's time to think about the first step: a surfing lesson. Although surfing lessons are a relatively recent phenomenon and it's totally possible to teach yourself to surf or get friends to teach you, going back to (surf) school is a great way to make the learning process easier and more fun.

Not only that, with so many girls wanting surf lessons now—in Australia an estimated 300,000 people take surf lessons every year and up to 70 percent are females—surf schools are responding to the increasing demand with girl-friendly options. There are all-girl surf schools, female surfing instructors, all-girl classes, and surf camps for women of all ages. Surf Diva in La Jolla, California, for instance, the world's first women's surf school when it opened its doors in 1996, is now America's largest, teaching up to five thousand girls to surf every year and employing about fifty female instructors every summer.

Why are so many girls taking surf lessons? According to Isabelle (Izzy) Tihanyi, co-founder and CEO of Surf Diva, they prefer a more structured approach when they're learning something new. "Women want to know everything and really feel comfortable before they get in the water," she says, "whereas guys want to learn to surf by doing it."

Beyond the practicalities of surfing, all-girl surf lessons can provide an encouraging and supportive environment. As Izzy explains, "I find that certain fears are really gender-based. A lot of women don't want to get in the way; that's a big fear. And we don't want to make fools of ourselves or upset anybody else—we're very concerned about other people and about not running over someone."

Surf lessons can also reduce the performance anxiety that accompanies any new activity. "People come to Surf Diva and say, 'Do you guarantee that I'll stand up?' and I say, 'No, but I'll guarantee that you'll have fun.' Women want to enjoy the process of learning. I like to compare it to getting ready for a party: Some-

SERENA BROOKE, PRO SURFER AND SURF COACH: It's a lot less intimidating learning at a surf school than trying to do it all by yourself, because you have someone giving you the tips you need and you get to surf with other girls at your level. And the instructors can show you what you're doing wrong, which is easier than correcting bad habits later.

times it's more fun to get ready—to figure out what you're going to wear and who you're going to go with—than to actually be there. The minute you take away that pressure to perform, women do better anyway, because there's less frustration, less anxiety."

Ultimately, whether you have surf lessons or not will depend on lots of variables: how you like to learn new things, how comfortable you feel in the ocean, whether you know any other surfers who are willing and able to teach you the basics. But think of it this way: What have you got to lose? Besides your dignity—and that won't last long whichever learn-to-surf path you choose!

Why go to surf school? The benefits of having lessons

- You'll learn the basics more quickly than if you were trying to teach yourself or learn from a friend. Plus, you'll get lots of tips and can break bad habits early on.
- You'll be shown where to surf, where to paddle out, and where to sit to catch waves.
- Surf schools supply surfboards, wetsuits, leashes, sunscreen, and insurance!
- It's fun! The more the merrier, right? Learning with other people (especially girls) at your level can be really comforting—you don't feel like the only one making a fool of yourself, you realize you're not alone, and it's just fun to be out in the water with other surfers at your level.
- You can try out different boards before buying one of your own, and get expert advice on which board or wetsuit suits you.
- It's safe. You're learning with qualified surf coaches who

GO-SURFING-WITH-OTHER-GIRLS DAYS

All-girl surf days can be a great introduction to surfing and a great way to meet other girl surfers in your area. The **Op Learn to Ride Days** are held in more than seventy-five locations throughout the United States and Canada every summer; **Roxy Surf Camps** (one-day surf camps for girls) happen along the West Coast starting in San Diego and ending in Santa Cruz, July to September; the **Billabong Summer Sessions Surf Camps Tour** travels along the East and West Coast in July with their all-star team, including Keala Kennelly, Belen Connelly, and Sanoe Lake; and the **Serena Brooke Days** are big in Florida and California. Some surf schools even hold their own all-girl surf days: Surf Academy runs an Annual Wild Woman Waterday at Surfrider Beach, Malibu, in August (see Appendix 3 for contact details).

know the beach intimately and can keep you away from local hazards such as rocks or rips. Plus, you get to learn about surf safety.

● You can take a lesson no matter what level you're at and you'll always learn something. No matter how much or how little surfing experience you have, when you go for a lesson your instructor will put you in a class that matches your level.

How to find a surf school that suits you

Surf schools come in all shapes and sizes: There are now more all-girl surf schools than ever before and many other surf schools have female surfing instructors and offer all-girl lessons and surf camps to make the learning-to-surf process more accessible for women (see Appendix 3 for contact details). And the offerings are more varied than ever before: from beginners' lessons (around $50 for a two-hour group lesson) to five-day surf camps and one-on-one coaching sessions.

Finding a reputable surf school is the easy part. Surfing America has a listing of all reputable surf schools and accredited surfing instructors and coaches (see Appendix 3 for contact details). Or ask about surf lessons at your local surf shop, and look for advertisements in newspapers and surfing magazines.

The next thing to do is decide on a lesson or program that suits your needs, budget, and available time:

● Do you want a private lesson, which is more expensive but provides more personal attention? Or a group lesson—more fun, cheaper, and you meet like-minded people but there's less personal attention?

● Do you want a morning lesson, when the waves have more chance of being clean and unruffled by the wind, or an afternoon one, when you might be feeling more awake and active?

● Try a one- or two-hour lesson if you just want to give surfing a go, or if you're not sure you're fit enough to surf longer, bearing in mind that part of that time will be spent on the beach. For a more intensive learning experience, there are overnight and weeklong surf camps. Some surf schools offer Monday-to-Friday surf clinics with a two-hour lesson each day. Or you might want to be creative: get together with a couple of friends and set up your own learn-to-surf schedule, such as a two-hour lesson every Saturday morning for a month.

IZZY TIHANYI, SURF DIVA SURF SCHOOL: We have people who have never even seen the ocean before—people coming from the Midwest or Canada or Europe—and learning to surf is a big deal for them. We taught some French girls recently and as they were paddling out, as soon as the wave hit them, they stood up facing *away* from the beach and tried to surf the wave *out* instead of *in*! They really had no concept of surfing.

What you can expect to learn in a two-hour lesson

As an example of what happens in a typical surf lesson, let's enroll ourselves in Surf Diva's most popular program for beginners aged 12 and over, the Level 1 Weekend Clinic. For $130 you get two 2-hour group lessons, one lesson on Saturday and one on Sunday. Wetsuits, soft-top surfboards, and sunscreen are all supplied; there are up to twelve students per class; and the instructor/student ratio is 1:5.

When you show up for your lesson, either at Surf Diva's headquarters in La Jolla, California, or one of their other locations, they'll give you a wetsuit and make sure it fits right, then you'll all stroll down to the beach, about a block away, where the surfboards are waiting. If you have surfed before, the lesson will consist mainly of revision of what you know, practice, and coaching from the instructor in the water. For first timers, the drill is:

● The instructors lead the group to a suitable spot on the beach and the lesson officially begins with introductions, a few stretches, and application of sunscreen (they supply it if anyone's forgotten to bring their own). Meeting your fellow students reminds you that you're not the only one feeling apprehensive or weird about learning to surf.

● Then comes a complete orientation to surfing: the instructors talk about water safety, surfing etiquette, how to avoid getting run over in the surf, how to avoid stepping on stingrays (a common hazard at La Jolla), and how to control your own board. Then you learn the parts of the surfboard, how to lie on your board, how to paddle, and how to catch waves—lying down at first, then standing up—and you practice pop-ups on the beach before heading into the water. This all takes about 45 minutes; on the second day the beach orientation only takes about 20 minutes, so you get to spend more time in the water.

● Next, everyone wades out into waist-deep water and practices lying on the boards, paddling, and catching the whitewater lying down. The first few times, your instructor might hold the back of your board to stabilize you or push you onto the waves, depending on the conditions.

● Surf Diva's instructors encourage you to get comfortable with your board first, by catching waves lying down, but when you feel that you can ride a wave and control your board, you can try to pop up. For the rest of the lesson you can practice catching waves, standing up, and riding them to the beach, with your instructor nearby giving you tips and plenty of encouragement. Of course you and your fellow "divas" will be offering encouragement to one another too!

● At the end of the lesson, everyone returns to the beach for a debrief: the instructors recap what you've learned and what to think about for the next lesson. Then you all stretch, drink lots of water to rehydrate, and walk back to the shop (the surfboards stay on the beach) with your new surfer friends.

What surf schools won't teach you

The bottom line with everything you learn, and this is particularly true in surfing, is that no matter how many lessons you have or how many tips you get from other surfers, the only one who can do it is you. It's you who has to get your board out in the water, paddle for those waves, and eventually stand up and ride them.

Surf schools also have limited time—sure, you can keep coming back for more lessons, but sooner or later you'll be on your own. That's not a bad thing, it's just the way surfing is. Unless you have a surf coach or friend watching your every move every time you surf, you're going to be spending a lot of time out in the water by yourself. And no matter how hopeless (and maybe helpless!) you might feel, one thing is guaranteed: Every time you get in the water, you're learning something. It might be something as simple as how the onshore wind makes the waves messy and harder to catch, how the waves get hollow and fast at low tide, or how to sit on your board without falling off.

You might be able to learn to stand up on a surfboard in a relatively short time, but learning about surfing—about the wind and weather, tides, surfing safely, the whole deal—is a lifelong journey.

How dangerous is surfing, really?

Because you're in a natural environment that has rhythms and rules all its own, surfing has its dangers, and when you're learning you need to be aware of them—not because you're more exposed to them (some of the worst injuries happen to experienced surfers) but because you often don't know what can happen.

The good news is that you're not alone in feeling scared or

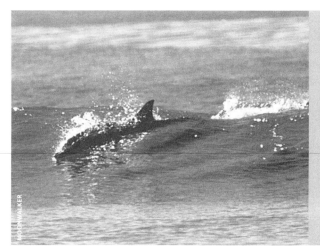

DO DOLPHINS REALLY REPEL SHARKS?

 It's a common misconception that seeing a pod of dolphins in the water means there aren't any sharks nearby. In fact the presence of dolphins can indicate that sharks are in the neighborhood too. Although dolphins have been known to help or warn humans in danger—and they are lovely to have around—both sharks and dolphins feed on fish. And big sharks, such as Great Whites, eat dolphins.

worried. In fact, it's good to be at least a little afraid; it means you're taking surfing seriously and respecting the ocean, and you'll be paying attention when you get out into the water, which is the single most important lesson you can learn.

According to Ross Phillips, surf coach and director of Surf Schools International, only four out of every thousand surfers will sustain some kind of injury requiring treatment—most commonly a strained muscle or being cut by a surfboard's fin. Compare that to about sixty-five per thousand for those playing soccer or football, he says, and surfing looks pretty safe!

That said, it's important to be aware of the potential dangers, how real they are, and what you can do to tiptoe around them.

What are you afraid of . . . sharks?

Let's get the big one out of the way first. The one with rows and rows of sharp pointy teeth and a big black dorsal fin that slices through the water just before it dives under your board and prepares to . . . *Hold it!*

Although, in theory, every time you enter the water you're back

ALISON: I don't really worry about sharks. I just think that, you know, I'm really big on grooming and I've had a shower very recently using a very nice Crabtree & Evelyn soap product, and there's fifteen boys out there who are peeing, at this very moment, in their wetsuits and probably haven't had a bath since September. They're going to smell so much more appealing to sharks than me!

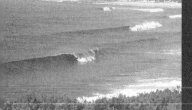

in the food chain, your actual chances of being eaten, or even nibbled, are relatively slim. As the people at the University of Florida's International Shark Attack File point out, you've got more chance of dying from a bee sting or snakebite (that's supposed to be comforting?).

Here's why your chances of being attacked by a shark are minimal:

● You're probably going to be surfing, at least when you're starting out, in urban areas where the beaches are patrolled by lifeguards who are only too happy to sound the alarm if a shark cruises by.

● The odds are in your favor. About 235 million people visit the beach every year, according to the U.S. Lifesaving Association, and in 2003 there were only 41 shark attacks across the whole country, over the whole year.

● Only a small percentage of shark attacks are fatal. That is, of the 41 unprovoked shark attacks in North America in 2003, only four were fatal. Most sharks attack surfers out of curiosity, and as soon as they take a bite out of your surfboard, they realize why surfers aren't on their everyday menu. Not only that, but unprovoked shark attacks worldwide have been decreasing for several years now. (All shark attack figures from the International Shark Attack File).

Besides all that, the more time you spend in the water, the more you develop your own unique survival instinct, so you'll be able to recognize when it feels safe to surf and when it doesn't. But for now, here are a few ways to minimize your chances of becoming a passing shark's next meal.

BETHANY HAMILTON, HAWAIIAN SURFER WHO LOST HER ARM IN A SHARK ATTACK IN OCTOBER 2003 AT AGE THIRTEEN, WHILE SURFING IN KAUAI: I was always scared of sharks and now even more, of course, but surfing is my life and I still get wet every day. To stay safe, surf with pals and always be alert, watch the bad weather and early mornings. And if you see a shark, catch a wave! Or at least lie still on your board and keep your arms and legs together!

Q: IS IT SAFE TO SURF DURING THAT TIME OF THE MONTH?

There's no conclusive evidence that menstrual blood attracts sharks, according to the International Shark Attack File. Most surfer girls I know, myself included, don't change their surfing habits to accommodate Shark Week, as one of them quaintly calls it—besides, the experience of surfing during your period more than makes up for any risks because it makes you feel good when you would otherwise be feeling crampy, bloated, or cranky! If you're worried, stay out of the water on the days of heaviest flow and always wear tampons when you surf during your period.

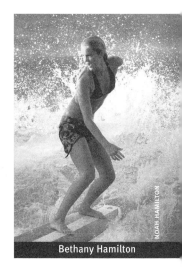
Bethany Hamilton

Ten ways to avoid being attacked by a shark:

1. Don't pee in your wetsuit. Urine is a sure sign of distress, and sharks respond to minute concentrations of urine the way tow-truck drivers respond to 911 calls.
2. Don't bleed into the water. If you cut yourself while surfing, paddle in. Sharks can detect one part blood in 25,000 parts of water more than half a mile from where you're innocently sitting on your board waiting for your last wave in.
3. Don't surf at dusk or before dawn; these are notorious shark-feeding times.
4. Don't surf near fishermen—where there's fishermen, there are fish scraps, and sharks, being natural scavengers, will probably be cruising in the vicinity.
5. Don't surf near river mouths. Although river mouths often get great waves because of the way the sand gets deposited as the water moves in and out of the river, they're also renowned shark hangouts because of the debris and assorted animal matter that often flows into the sea from farther upstream.
6. Keep your dog out of the water. Dogs attract sharks by their activity—in the water and at the water's edge—and by their scent.
7. Don't surf at night. Sounds obvious, but you'd be surprised how desperate you can get when you have to deal with crowded city surf beaches! Seriously, though, you can find yourself in the water very late in the day when you're trying to get that elusive last wave in. Try not to be the last one out of the water, and paddle in to the beach if you have to.
8. If you see a shark, don't panic. Try to put your board between it and you, hit it on the nose (sharks are extra sensitive there), and paddle to the beach as fast as you can.
9. Surf with a friend. Sharks are more likely to attack a lone surfer than someone surfing in a group.
10. Don't hum the theme from *Jaws* or talk about sharks while you're surfing. It might not attract sharks, but it will freak you out!

. . . other ocean nasties?

Just when you thought it was safe to go back in the water, there are a few other marine creatures to be wary of when you're surfing:

● **Man-o-wars** (also called Portuguese man-of-war or bluebottle): A summertime hazard on the East Coast, particularly in

Florida, and in Hawaii, man-o-wars are easily recognized by a blue-green bubble floating on the surface and a trailing bunch of long stinging tentacles that, if they come into contact with bare skin, will give you a nasty sting. Nothing life-threatening, but it does hurt and can itch for days afterward. Treatment: remove the tentacles and rinse with freshwater. Summer's onshore winds also bring sea nettles (a kind of jellyfish) and hatches of sea lice that, although they don't hurt, can drive you mad and force you to run to shore and strip off your rash guard and wetsuit!

● **Stingrays:** Usually found at beaches with relatively calm, warm water, stingrays can inflict severe pain with the barbed spines in their whiplike tails. To avoid stepping on them, do the "stingray shuffle" (shuffle your feet along the sandy bottom when you're walking in the water). If you are stung (usually on the foot), consult the lifeguards and immerse your foot in hot water.

● **Kelp:** This thick seaweed is a blessing for West Coast surfers because it keeps the surface of the water glassy, making the waves smooth and lovely to ride. It can become a hazard, however, if you or your leash get tangled in it.

● **Sea urchins:** These small, spiky balls of trouble are most commonly found in the crevices of rock platforms, especially in tropical surf locations like Hawaii. Step on one and the spines can stick into your bare feet and cause considerable agony. There's no venom in the spines, but they can be tricky to remove, so if you have tender tootsies consider getting a pair of wetsuit booties to wear when you surf in sea urchin–infested places.

● **Sharp coral:** Another hazard to bare feet (and other exposed body parts that come in contact with it in Hawaii and other tropical surf destinations) is coral. If you are grazed or cut by coral, rinse the wound immediately and apply antiseptic; cuts can quickly become infected, turning your surfing vacation into a laze-by-the-hotel-pool vacation.

. . . being hit by your surfboard?

When you're riding a board that's bigger and heavier than you are, it's natural to be scared of it. I know friends who, as competent bodysurfers, would brave waves of any size, but as soon as they

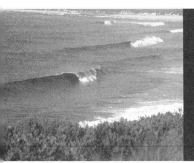

PRUE JEFFRIES, PRO SURFER: Surfing's not really a fear-based sport, it's more about surrender—it's like I'm going out into something that's bigger and more powerful than me and the only thing I can really do is learn to understand what's going on enough to take care of myself and go with the flow. I think girls are afraid they're going to get hit by their boards and cut up. It's just a matter of taking precautions and if you have a fear, then address it—take steps toward reducing it.

started surfing they freaked out at the thought of this big thing attached to their ankle.

I'd be lying if I said you couldn't get hit by your surfboard, but there are ways to avoid it. Try to get used to being aware of where your board is (and possibly other surfers' boards), where it's going to go, and where you are in relation to it. And although the kind of board you'll be learning on is bigger than your basic shortboard, be thankful that it has a rounded (not pointy) nose.

How to avoid being clobbered by your board (or someone else's):

● When you're walking out into the surf, always keep your board beside or behind you; make sure your board isn't between you and the oncoming waves.

● Don't paddle out behind another surfer; although in theory they should look behind them if they lose their board, it's you who's going to get injured if their board washes onto you so it's your responsibility to stay out of the way.

● When you wipe out, always put your arms over your head and face to protect them in case you surface under your board or your board springs back at you after you've come up. And try to stay underwater until you can't feel your board straining against you anymore.

● Try to fall off behind your board, or fall into the whitewater of the wave, not in front of the wave.

If the possibility of hitting your board is really worrying you, always surf with someone else or try learning on a softboard—they're made out of the same materials as bodyboards and have soft rubber fins that won't cut you. Most surf schools use softboards for these very reasons. (More about all kinds of surfboards in Chapter 3.)

. . . getting hurt?

Surfboards are scary-looking things. They have three sharp fins at the back; a leash that can get snagged on rocks, wrapped around your legs, or, worse, your neck; and when surfboards are damaged, the fiberglass splinters can be razor sharp. Not only that, shortboards have ridiculously pointy noses that can take out an eye (yours or someone else's). Prevention: If your fins are ultra sharp, get some sandpaper and smooth them down a bit. If you ride a shortboard, buy a nose guard and stick it to the pointy nose of your board as soon as you can. When you wipe out, always try to fall away from your board, particularly if it looks like it's going to land with the fins up.

Waves can of course be dangerous too. Surf spots all over the world have notoriously scary names—like Crackneck, Lacerations, Hospitals, Voodoo, Boneyards, and Scar Reef—and for good reason: They can hurt you. Wipe out over sharp coral reef or urchin-encrusted rocks, and you may have to stay out of the water for weeks to let your injuries heal. Often, the best way to avoid getting hurt is just to respect your limits and know where you can (and can't) safely surf.

The flip side to getting hurt in the surf, however, is one that you often don't realize until you're having to explain to your loved ones how you got that massive cut in your leg/arm/head: your first surf injury is a rite of passage. Someone once told me that scars are better than tattoos because they have more interesting stories—and surf injuries definitely do. Even if you wiped out, a surf injury is a mark of honor, an initiation—because you were out there, having an adventure in a potentially risky environment.

. . . water pollution?

Toxic water is, sadly, a fact of life at many of our beaches these days, particularly after heavy rain when stormwater drains overflow and disgorge their contents into the ocean. Wastewater treatment plants can also become overloaded by the increased volume of water, and surfers are generally the ones who suffer the outcome: raw sewage, debris, and other pollutants floating around the lineup, causing everything from ear and eye infections to more serious illnesses such as hepatitis.

The simplest solution is to stay out of the water for a few days

ANGIE:
When I got my first fin chop [cut from a surfboard fin], I was so stoked I showed everyone! My first fin chop was more a mark of pride than a wound. It shows that you've really been in the elements.

after heavy rain or whenever you suspect the water is polluted. But that's easier said than done because the weather patterns that bring rain often bring waves too (more on this in Chapter 4).

So what can you do? Use your common sense. If the water looks murky or littered with debris, wait until the wind goes off-shore and the wave action cleans up the conditions. Ask the local lifeguards or rangers when it's safe to go in the water. Of course, if you have any open cuts or wounds or if you're just feeling run-down, it'd be wise to stay out of the water for a bit longer than you otherwise would. Rinsing your ears and eyes in fresh water immediately after surfing can be a good idea too.

For water quality updates, ask your local surf shop or lifeguard. The Surfrider Foundation and Beach.com monitor water quality at beaches in California, Hawaii, Texas, Florida, and Alabama (with more coastal states to be included soon). Heal the Bay also issues weekly Beach Report Cards for more than 430 California beaches, and their website lists California beaches when they are closed due sewage-related spills (see Appendix 3 for contact details).

Looking longer-term, you can try to minimize the part you play in water pollution. Be aware that whatever goes on the roads or down your kitchen sink ends up in the ocean. Wash your car on grass, not on the road. Pick up any rubbish on your street. Don't put anything down your kitchen (or bathroom or laundry) sink that you wouldn't want to see next time you paddle out. Use ocean-friendly cleaning products. Don't let plastic bags escape your home; take a cloth bag with you when you shop or ask for (biodegradable) paper bags instead of plastic ones. Think of it as a thank-you to the ocean for all the waves you're going to be surfing soon!

When you start surfing more, your local beach becomes an extension of your backyard and as surfers we can set a good example.

. . . fear itself?

Welcome to the mental dimension of surfing, namely, your mind and its handmaidens: fears and insecurities. Even if you think you don't have any (or many!), surfing will find them for you. Maybe it's a fear of surfing alone or surfing at dusk; maybe it's a fear of sharks or of being knocked unconscious by your own board . . . sometimes just being around waves that are bigger than you can freak you out. The important thing is to realize that fear is a natural response to an unfamiliar environment, and most surfers experience fear at some time during their surfing lives, if not all the time!

I've thought about fear a lot when I've found myself out of my comfort zone and watched other surfers taking off on waves that scared the daylights out of me. Are they just not afraid? Or do they have the same fear as I have and do it anyway? I might never know the answer, but I do know that some fear is healthy—it keeps you alert when you need to be, makes sure you're aware of what's going on around you. It's also what makes surfing exciting—that surge of adrenaline you get when you survive a situation you thought was beyond you is one fantastic feeling.

Perhaps the thing to remember is that when your fear levels get so high that you feel unable to do anything, it might be time to head back to the beach. Also, the point at which you feel fear will shift: The situations that scare you today might not scare you next week. Sometimes when you're feeling strong, you'll be more confident, and when you haven't surfed for a while you'll feel timid again. Just go with it and try to understand your own rhythms, so you know when to go surfing and when to hang back and watch from the safety of the shore.

Fear can also be useful, by letting you know what you have to work on. Maybe you're afraid of getting held under. If that's true for you, you could try doing some fitness training and practice holding your breath longer. Or maybe you're afraid of big waves, in which case it's a good idea to go and watch them whenever you can, to familiarize yourself with them without putting your safety on the line. That will make them seem easier to handle when you're out in them the next time.

. . . rips and currents?

There'll be more on rips later (in Chapter 6), but for now it's good to know a couple of things about these seemingly scary obstacles to your surfing success.

Rips are currents that move directly away from the beach. Contrary to popular belief, though, they rarely go all the way out to sea. They usually stop just where the farthest-breaking waves are, which is why surfers use them to paddle out. Most rips are less than 30 feet wide and lose their power once they get to the line of breaking waves out the back.

The reason they have such a dangerous reputation is that if you get caught in a rip when you're swimming, you can get tired by struggling against its pull, be swept out of your depth and not know how (or be able) to get back to the beach. To get out of a rip, the trick is to swim diagonally across it (not against it). You can even let the rip take you out beyond the breakers, swim parallel to the beach, and then swim in through the surf zone.

When you're on a surfboard, rips aren't nearly as scary as they are when you're swimming. For one thing, you've got your board to keep you afloat, so if you do get caught in a rip, try to relax and either float with it until you get out the back, or paddle diagonally across it; then paddle in through the surf zone or let some breaking waves carry you in. The biggest problem with rips is when you inadvertently try to paddle in to the beach while you're in one—because rips occur where there are deep channels, there won't be any waves breaking to carry you to the shore, plus you'll be struggling against a current that's heading out to sea. If this happens to you, try to paddle sideways out of the rip and then find a breaking wave to carry you in.

A few cheerful facts about rips

- Rips occur when water that's been pushed toward the beach by waves needs to get back to the sea. They're natural phenomena, not the freakish disasters they're often made out to be.
- Because they're affected by the tide and other factors, rips can start and finish and move around without warning. Always be aware of the conditions when you're in the water.
- Rips can occur anywhere there's a channel that's deeper than the surrounding sandbars. For instance, wherever there's a headland and water has scoured a channel out of the sand just beside it, chances are there'll be a rip there (great for paddling out).
- You can spot a rip by the color of the water—it'll either be darker, because the water's deeper in a rip than on either side of it, or sandy, because the rip's carrying sand away from the beach. Waves will often be breaking on either side of the rip but not in the rip. And the water surface might be choppy in a rip, compared to either side of it.

. . . other surfers?

Whether we like it or not, the surfing environment is a male-dominated one, but being female in this "boy zone" has both advantages and disadvantages.

On the one hand, you're not as likely to cop much open aggression from guy surfers in the water: They'd be ridiculed by their friends for attacking a girl. But there are guys who hold firmly to the belief that, because you're female, you can't surf as well as they can. So they don't take any notice when you're paddling for a wave they want; they'll either paddle around you, or over the top of you, or blatantly steal the wave from you. It's up to you to let them know that's not okay. Even if you're a beginner, you're still entitled to your fair share of waves. If someone looks like they're going to take your wave, just call out "Yep" or something else you can say clearly and at short notice; hopefully when they see you're up and riding the wave quite capably (or at least giving it a go), they'll back off and wait for a wave of their own.

The advantage of being female in the lineup is that guys often give you the benefit of the doubt. They'll forgive you for blunders like "dropping in" (more about this in Chapter 8). Some guys will call you onto waves simply because you're a girl and might not be getting as many waves as the guys out there. Most guys are keen to see more girls in the surf and give you encouragement whenever they can. Don't abuse such special treatment, appreciate it.

There's something else about the female presence out in the water. There are aggressive female surfers, but most girls are out there to have fun, not to prove themselves. I've even heard guys say that when a girl paddles out into the lineup, everyone relaxes a bit. And it's amazing what an icebreaker a big smile can be.

The embarrassment factor (or "Does my butt look big in this wetsuit?")

There's one more issue that plagues a lot of females learning to surf: feeling self-conscious about the way you look when you're in the water, feeling like an idiot for getting hammered by every wave that comes your way, and being pretty confident that you look like a drowned rat in the process.

Believe it or not, there are fashion advantages to surfing, apart from all the cool surf gear you can wear on land. Sure, wetsuits are more revealing than anything you'd generally wear in public, but at least they're in slimming black! Besides, no one on the beach can see you when you're in the water. In summer you get to wear baggy boardshorts. And I don't want to spoil the surprise but the more you surf, the less you'll actually care about how other people see you. You'll be having too much fun!

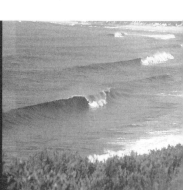

ANGIE: There is an embarrassment barrier, but you just have to get over it. A friend of mine once said to me when I was first surfing, "Mate, while you're walking on the beach to the surf and when you're walking back, nobody has any idea. They could be thinking, Wow, she's just had the best surf of her life." They have no idea that you've been out there just being tumbled by every single wave that came in! So he said, "Just smile and walk by and think, I can do this, I'm a surfer!" That's always stuck in my head because even when I have a bad surf, I just think, Those guys weren't here before, they probably think I rip it up!

Surfing, it'll change your life—or at least your body

Wondering how surfing will change you? Put simply, surfing sculpts your body in subtle ways. Unlike swimming, it makes you strong without giving you beefy shoulders. It gives your arms definition and brings out your triceps, the muscles at the back of your arms that are responsible for your paddling.

Then there's the rest of your body. Surfing's great for your general fitness. There's the aerobic exercise of paddling out and around the break. Springing to your feet when you stand up on your board tones your thighs. Sitting and balancing on your board tones your stomach and sides. Paddling and sitting on your board, and also turning your board and twisting, strengthens your back. Walking on the sand even exfoliates your feet!

And because you're having so much fun doing it, you often don't realize how much exercise you're getting. Plus, you're breathing sea air and you're in the ocean—and that has multiple positive effects on your general sense of well-being.

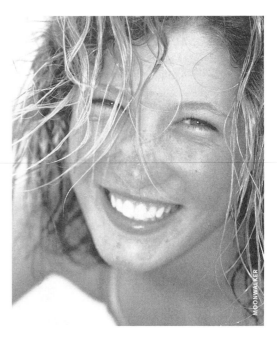

✳ Surfing bleaches your hair, freckles your nose, browns your body, and puts a smile on your face!

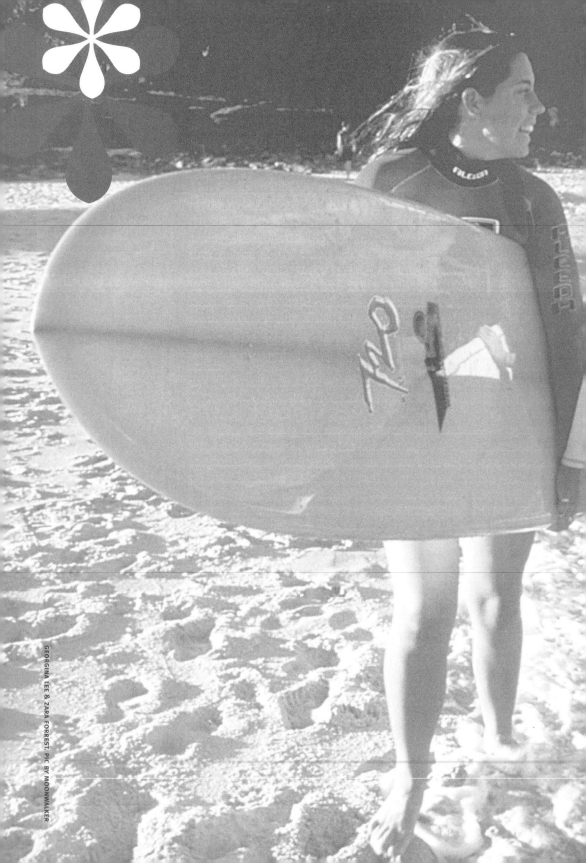

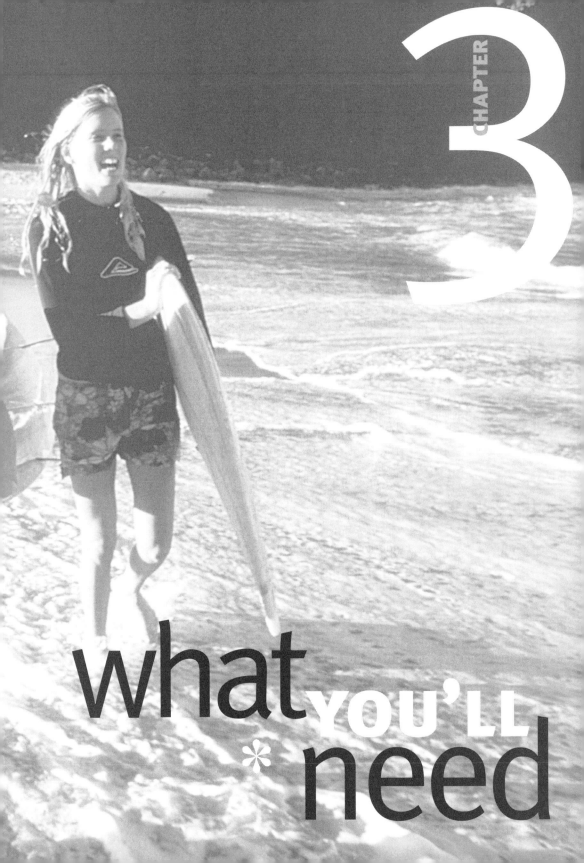

what you'll * need

Learn:

How to **choose** your **first** surfboard. What your options are: softboards, **fiberglass** boards, plastic boards. **Board-buying tips.** What to **wear** in the surf: all about **bikinis**, boardshorts, rash guards, wetsuits. **Other gear you'll need: leashes, wax and deck grip, surfboard bags, sun protection, nose guards, booties, helmets, ding repair kits, and roof racks.**

O ne of the best things about surfing is that it's relatively inexpensive. The waves are free, after all. And the wind that creates them, and the tides, and . . . wait a minute! Although surfers are renowned minimalists, we do need some equipment. Most important of all is the surfboard.

The right board

Just as surfers come in all shapes and sizes, so do surfboards. Although people have been known to ride all kinds of crazy craft— I once saw a guy in Indonesia surfing on a piece of wood—this chapter deals with boards that you can ride standing up. There are other ways to surf: kneeling (on a kneeboard), lying down (on a bodyboard or surf mat), or sitting (on a surf kayak). You might find that one of these suits you better than stand-up surfing, but it's a good idea to start with the generic form of surfing and go from there.

There are two basic kinds of surfboards: longboards and short-boards. **Shortboards** are basically pointy-nosed surfboards that are under 7 feet long. They're best suited to surfers with a bit of experience, since they are lighter and less stable than big, gentle longboards and are easier to turn so you can throw them around a bit more. Because they're so light, you need to ride the steepest, most critical part of the wave, which is why they're for experienced surfers. Virtually all shortboards have three fins.

Longboards generally start around 7 foot 6 inches in length. Their rounded noses and considerable bulk make them ideal for learning; the extra volume gives them more flotation so you can catch waves more easily (that is, with less effort). Longboards have either one large fin, often accompanied by two smaller side fins, or three fins of equal size. The very first surfers rode longboards, and they're still the best boards to learn on. Why?

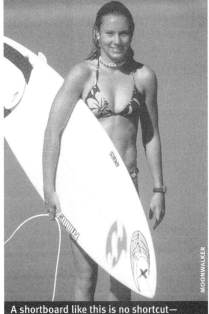

- Because they float so well, they're easy to paddle and allow you to catch waves with the least amount of effort.
- Because of their Battlestar Galactica size, they're more stable, and therefore easier to lie, sit, and stand up on.
- You can catch waves before they get too steep; this gives you time to stand up and get your balance before the ride really begins.
- You can catch smaller (and therefore safer) waves.

A shortboard like this is no shortcut—
bigger is better for beginners

What kind of board do I need?

For your very first surfboard, your best bet is a **mini-longboard**, which is a longboard between 7 and 9 feet long with a rounded nose and three fins. These are the basic prerequisites for your first board. Don't worry about specifying thickness or rails—most boards are in proportion to their length.

Although you need a board between 7 and 9 foot, the ideal **length** for you will depend on your height, weight, fitness, and general enthusiasm. As a basic rule of thumb, go for a shorter board if you're shorter, fitter, and going to be surfing a lot. If you're going to be surfing every day as opposed to only surfing on the weekends, for example, you'll be able to use a shorter surfboard because your fitness will develop more quickly. One guideline that's often used for board length is this: stand with one arm raised over your head. Your ideal first board should be at least as long as you and your outstretched arm.

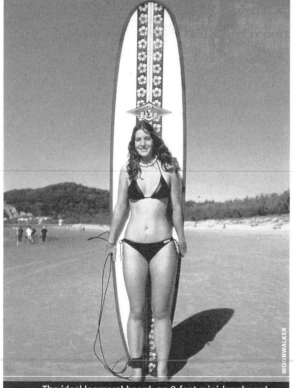

The ideal learners' board, an 8-foot mini-longboard

The trick is to get a board that's big enough for you to paddle easily and stand on, while still light enough for you to carry, paddle out through white-water, and (eventually!) turn.

You also want a board with a **wide rounded nose**, not a narrow pointy nose. A wide nose means there's more volume (more board) to the front of the surfboard, which makes it easier to catch fuller, gentler waves. With pointy-nosed boards you generally have to catch waves at their steepest and most critical stage—not ideal when you're learning.

You also want the board to be fairly thick. A **thicker board** will keep you afloat more easily and, when you're floating on the surface, rather than sinking into the water, the board will be easier to paddle. It'll also catch waves more easily. Think of a piece of wood floating around in the surf. If it's light and floaty, the waves will just pick it up and carry it to shore!

Finally, your first board needs

three fins. Some longboards have a big center fin and two smaller side fins, but what you want is three fins of equal size, because that's what you'll probably be riding when you progress from your first board. Whether you decide to head into shortboard territory or go for a "real" longboard (at least 9 feet long), most boards these days have three fins, because they're easier to turn. Single-fin boards can be more stable and although that is an advantage when you're starting out, the real joy of surfing comes when you learn to turn.

Can I learn to surf on a shortboard?

The conventional wisdom is that shortboards aren't the best learn-to-surf boards, simply because they're too unstable and harder to paddle than longboards. Having said that, sometimes a shortboard *can* be better to learn on:

● Kids often learn to surf really easily on shortboards because kids are light and agile. They don't need the stability of a longer board. A good rule of thumb is: The older and less athletic you are, the longer the board you need.
● Some shortboards are as thick as a longboard—so what you lose in length you make up for in thickness.
● If you're a natural athlete, competent snowboarder or skater, and really fit, you might get away with learning on a shortboard because you already have great balance and board skills.

If you do decide to learn on a shortboard, do yourself a favor and make sure it has three fins—single-fin surfboards are less stable and harder to turn. Most important, don't go for just any old shortboard. Get some solid advice from someone you trust. And beware the well-meaning friends who say, "Yeah, you can have that old six-foot twin-fin under the house; it'd be perfect for you!" It won't be—and it might force you to give up surfing before you even get started.

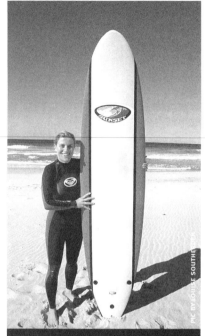

Esther and Sunset softboard showing top . . .

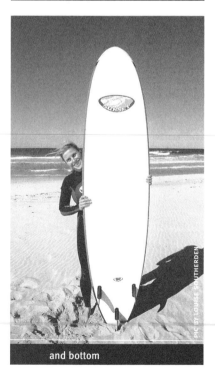

and bottom

The options

There's a huge array of options for the first-time surfer these days. According to John Radcliffe, owner of Dripping Wet Surf Company in Manly Beach, Sydney, "People now have access to much better equipment: it's cheaper, there's a lot more acceptance of beginners, there's legropes [leashes] and wetsuits. . . . I learned on a 9'10" longboard because there was nothing else. It was ugly and I could never carry it. I had trouble catching waves because I kept getting washed back, and when I did stand up on it, there was no way I could turn it because it only had one fin. I hated that board. The only reason I kept surfing was because Mum and Dad surfed. The best thing that happened was when it broke and my dad and I trimmed two feet off the end of it, and made it a 7'10"! And there were no wetsuits when I learned—I used to wear a woolen jumper, can you believe that? It's a wonder I never drowned!"

Here's the lowdown on your three main options:

- Softboards
- Plastic boards
- Fiberglass boards

Softboards

Softboards are basically surfboards made out of bodyboard materials—polyethylene foam with a white plastic bottom, a stringer for strength, and "real" plastic fins—and they come in lots of cool colors. There are several brands, including Doyle, Sunset, BZ, and Szabad, which all retail for $300 to $400.

Because they're not as hard as regular fiberglass boards and have soft rubber fins, softboards make a great first board if you're concerned about getting hurt or injuring someone else. They're also reasonably immune to unsightly (and water-absorbing) dings. Most surf schools use softboards, and surf shops often rent them out for about $20 per day, so you can try before you buy.

The disadvantage of these boards is their performance: They just don't move through the water or turn as easily as fiberglass or even plastic boards. This might make them easier to ride initially, but you'll outgrow their easy learning curves sooner rather than later.

They're also pretty heavy—heavier than fiberglass boards of the same size—which can make them a hassle to carry to and from the beach or to lift onto the roof racks of your car.

Plastic boards

Plastic (or pop-out) surfboards are light and extremely durable and perform better than softboards for around the same price: an NSP plastic board will set you back about $350 to $500, depending on its length. Their main advantage is that they're tough, so you can concentrate on your surfing instead of worrying about keeping your brand-new surfboard ding-free.

On the downside, because they're mass produced, plastic boards are pretty crudely shaped, so you're less likely to find one that suits your build and surfing style. And, again, you'll probably outgrow it as soon as you can stand up and go along a wave. A not-too-distant cousin of the plastic board is the epoxy surfboard. Lightweight and durable, they can be stiff and almost too buoyant; they're also usually too expensive to be a realistic option as a first board.

Fiberglass boards

Most surfers, beginners or otherwise, ride fiberglass surfboards for the simple reason that they're lightweight and move well through the water. They can also be made to measure (see next page). Fiberglass surfboards are actually made of foam, like Styrofoam, which is then covered with fiberglass cloth and coated with resin to seal it. They have a wooden stringer down the center for added strength; without a stringer, the board would need to have a thicker, heavier coating of resin to keep it from breaking whenever there was any impact on it, such as the lip of a breaking wave. The stringer allows the board to be strong yet lightweight and therefore more maneuverable.

The great thing about a fiberglass board is that you'll probably want to hang on to it long after you move to your next surfboard, because they're really fun to ride, particularly in small waves. They're

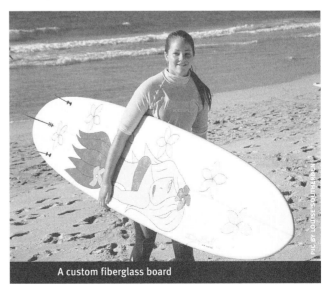

A custom fiberglass board

KAITLYN: When I first started surfing I was a complete and total mess. I couldn't stay up on the board, mostly because I was on my dad's, which was 6'8" with a pointed front and was so hard to handle. Now I'm riding a 7'3" Bic [plastic] board, which is much sturdier. I can get up on it easier, and I really love the way it handles: it's very stable but it's also easy to turn, and it's tough!

also cheaper, lighter, and more readily available and perform better than soft or plastic boards.

The disadvantages? They hurt when they hit you, and they get dinged and need repairing with resin. (If left unrepaired, the dings can let water into the absorbent foam core of the board, or their sharp edges can cut you.)

New or used?

This really depends on your budget. The trick is to spend enough to get a board that's good for you to learn on, while not spending too much, because it's probably going to get dinged, and you'll want to replace it when you outgrow it.

Beginners often buy used boards because they don't want to damage a perfect new board; it's less heartbreaking to ding a board that's already got a few injuries! But if you can get a new board for the same price, go for it; it's a great feeling to walk out of a shop and onto the beach with a shiny new board that no one has ever ridden.

Made to measure

You can even go a step further and order a custom-made surfboard. While this might seem extravagant for your first surfboard (custom boards often cost a little more than surfboards bought off the rack from a surf shop), learning to surf on a board that is designed specifically for you will really speed up the learning process.

You don't have to know what you want (or need) to get a great custom board; that's the shaper's job. One shaper who has spent several years trying to understand what beginner surfer girls need is Shawn Ambrose of Trixie Surfboards in Oceanside, California. "When I first started making surfboards for girls, I had the same opinion a lot of shapers did: put the girls on a bigger board. Then I started rethinking everything, and over the last four years I've come up with the Supermodel, which is our ultimate beginner's board."

If you start with a basic shape like the Supermodel, you can then have it tailor-made to suit your height, weight, build, and surfing ability. But whether you go ready-made or made-to-order, it helps to know a few features to look for when you're scouting around for your first board. To give you a head start, here are the essential ingredients of the Trixie Surfboards Supermodel: It's wide enough to be stable but narrow enough to get your arm around to carry it (girls tend to have narrower shoulders than guys) and narrow enough to maneuver (we have smaller feet too). It has a bit of curve in the nose to keep it from nose-diving when you take off on a wave and to allow you to angle across the wave. It also has a narrower tail than a standard beginner's board to make it easier to turn, so you don't outgrow it when your surfing progresses.

What's it going to cost?

Surfing is one of the most reasonably priced activities around. The board is going to be your main expense: They start at around $150 to $200 for a decent used mini-longboard, and around $300 to $400 for a brand new mini-longboard, usually including a leash.

But there are ways to minimize costs (remember, surfers are the ultimate minimalists): borrow a friend's board while you're learning, rent a board every time you go out or ask someone who loves you to help you buy a surfboard for your next birthday!

Try before you buy

Renting surfboards is one of the best ways to get a feel for the type and size of board you need. When you rent a board from your local surf shop, tell them what level you're at and how much you've surfed, and ask them what size they'd recommend. They'll probably give you a softboard (the perfect learner's board), but ask to try out a few sizes and see what difference it makes. The biggest factor is length: longer boards are easier to stand up on but harder to carry and handle in the water.

How to buy a surfboard

When you're starting out, you're going to need all the help and advice you can get. The trick is in knowing who to trust. Surf schools are a great source of independent advice on what kind of board to buy. Not only do you get to try out a board thoroughly during the lesson but you can ask your instructor what kind of board would suit you.

Surf shops are your next port of call. But be warned: not all surf shops were created equal. Try to go to one where you feel comfortable—they might have music you like, surfing videos on the in-store TV, a good vibe about the place. Pick one that's girl-friendly, not oozing machismo. Most important, the people who work there should be experienced surfers who are friendly and helpful.

If someone's genuinely trying to sell you the right board for you

*tip

Be honest, not modest! Don't downplay what you have achieved in your surfing but don't exaggerate your ability either, or you could end up with the wrong board. Surfing's hard enough without handicapping yourself with a board that's not suited to you.

68

DO GIRLS AND GUYS NEED DIFFERENT SURFBOARDS?

The short answer is no, your ability and physical size are more important than your gender when it comes to choosing a surfboard that's right for you. On the other hand, it's a great feeling to ride a surfboard that's been especially shaped for a girl, as Izzy Tihanyi of Surf Diva surf school explains. "We have a line of Surf Diva women's surfboards shaped by veteran shaper Craig Hollingsworth made specifically for girls: they're narrower so a girl can carry them, they have great graphics, and they're made proportionate for smaller people. Guys can ride them, of course, but it's just like blue jeans: you can wear your boyfriend's jeans and they'll look great, but there's nothing better than a pair of jeans cut just for a girl."

(as opposed to the board they want to get rid of or the board they're going to make the most commission on), they're going to ask you as many questions as they can to find out where you're at with your surfing and who you are as a person. It's not enough that they know you're a beginner. To find your perfect board they'll need a bit more info, and you can help by telling them about yourself and being prepared for questions such as:

- Have you ever been on a surfboard before? What kind? Did you stand up?
- Have you ever had a lesson? What board did you ride, and did you like it? Did it feel too big, too short, too unstable? Was it too heavy for you to carry down to the water?
- Do you play any other sports? (This will help them assess your level of fitness.)
- How often do you think you'll be going surfing? (If you're committed to surfing a few times a week, rather than once every two weeks, you'll progress faster and probably need a lighter or shorter board.)

Finally, ask if there's any kind of guarantee. If you're not happy with a board you've bought, you should be able to go back and talk to the people who sold it to you. Although some shops are unscrupulous and won't want to see you again once you've waltzed out of their store with a new board under your arm, most shops want you to love your first surfboard so that you grow to love surfing and become a good customer throughout your surfing life. Reputable surf shops will always try to help, either by exchanging a board you don't like for one that might suit you better or allowing you to try a few different-sized boards before you commit to one.

Board-buying tips

● Take a friend with you. Shopping's always more fun with friends, and surfboard shopping's no different. Make sure your friend surfs, has seen you surf (if you have surfed before, that is), and knows the kind of board you're looking for.

● Be honest about how you surf and how often you're going to surf, what kind of waves you like, what your style is like, and what stage you're up to—for example, are you riding the whitewater, trying to stand up, skimming across green waves, doing lots of turns?

● Try not to be influenced by the board's color or artwork. Sure, you gotta love your board, but it's the shape that's going to help you surf better, not the color. Besides, your first board won't be with you forever; heartless as this might sound, one day you're going to outgrow its chunky curves. Go for dimensions, not looks.

● To see how it feels, hold the board under your arm as if you're walking down to the beach, and check that you can get your arm around it.

● If you're buying a fiberglass board, check for dings, particularly around the nose and tail. Beware of dings that have started to go brown—that means water has seeped into the board, which will make it heavy and less buoyant. Check for cracks on the rails that can let in water, creases (lines across the board where it's been stressed), and repaired breaks (they might make the board more vulnerable to breaking again).

● Check that the fins are solid by wiggling them a bit, and check for cracks in the resin at their base. If the board has removable fins (such as FCS fins), check for crusty salt around the plugs—that means salt water has entered the plugholes and possibly the board (not a good thing).

● When you find the board you want, don't be afraid to ask the shop to throw in a free leash and a bar of surf wax. Ask them to show you how to wax your board, attach your leash, and, if your board has removable ones, put in the fins.

What to wear?

Like any subculture, surfing has a range of outfits, although these are dictated more by practicality than appearance, and black (for wetsuits at least) is always in! What you'll be wearing depends on where you live, how much you feel the cold, how long you stay in the water in an average session, how many waves you usually catch (you stay warmer when you're paddling around, catching lots of waves than when you're sitting out the back waiting for the good ones), and what time of day you'll be surfing (it's cooler in the early morning and late afternoon than in the middle of the day).

Chances are you'll be learning to surf in summer and, unless you live somewhere like Northern California (or Canada!) where the water is always cold, you can basically get by with the bare (so to speak) minimum—bikini, boardshorts, and a rash guard—and expand your range to include wetsuits as the need arises.

Bikinis. Surfing in just a bikini—no rash guard, no board-shorts—is one of the best feelings known to woman. But there's a reason you don't see every surfer girl out there in a triangle top and bottom: They're hard to keep on in the surf. If your butt hits the wave, you get an instant thong. And if you wipe out, you can lose the top altogether. One-piece swimsuits get around this problem, but they're harder to change in and out of after your surf, and the bottom still rides up if you wipe out. The solution? Try to get a bikini that fits you really well and feels comfortable. Halter tops stay on better when you're paddling than bra-style tops. Personally, I'm always wary of bikinis with "optional extras" like beads or cute little rings or even ties at the side; they can become really uncomfortable when you're lying on your board or wearing them under a wetsuit. Boy-leg bikini bottoms are often more comfortable than boardshorts, and they reduce the embarrassment factor when you paddle past a bunch of prepubescent males! And of course you can team your bikini with a rash guard or a pair of boardshorts or both!

Rash guards. Also known as a rash vest or rash shirt, this is a Lycra T-shirt that was originally designed to be worn inside out

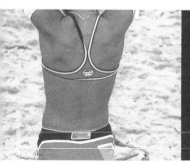

underneath your wetsuit to keep it from giving you a rash under your arms when you paddle. But wetsuits are now made of such soft neoprene, and often lined with Lycra as well, that rash guards are becoming increasingly unnecessary under them. They're still great for sun protection, however. You can also get rash guards that are warmer than just Lycra; Rip Curl's Hot Skins have a silver lining that reflects your body heat back to you instead of letting it escape.

When you're buying a rash guard, make sure it fits snugly all over—it's not supposed to be as loose as an ordinary T-shirt because it will get even looser when it's wet, and you want it to stay with you when you're paddling (when a rash guard gets old and loose, it can actually give you a rash).

Wetsuits. Unless you live in Hawaii or southern Florida, sooner or later you're going to need a wetsuit. Most wetsuits are made of a material called neoprene, which consists of a layer of rubber sandwiched between two layers of nylon fabric. Contrary to popular belief, it's not the rubber that keeps you warm but the layer of water trapped between the neoprene and your skin; your body heat warms the water, which insulates you from the cold. That's why it's important that your wetsuit fit well, particularly around your neck, wrists, and ankles.

Most wetsuits are described in terms of two numbers: the first number refers to the wetsuit's thickness on the legs and body (thicker rubber for extra warmth), the second refers to the thickness on the arms (thinner rubber for ease of movement). So a 3/2 fullsuit, for instance, has 3mm neoprene on the body and legs, and 2mm on the arms.

In case you're wondering, a fullsuit is a wetsuit with long sleeves and long legs, usually worn in winter (unless you live on the West Coast anywhere north of Santa Barbara, then you'll probably be wearing a fullsuit all year round). The other main styles of wetsuit are:

- Spring suits: short sleeves and short legs, usually only 2 mm thick. So named because they're usually worn between seasons when it's not cold enough for a fullsuit but too cold to surf without a wetsuit altogether.
- Long-armed spring suits: long sleeves, short legs. Warmer than a spring suit, without going all the way to a fullsuit. Usually made of lightweight neoprene, about 2 mm all over for ease of movement. As Todd Leetch from Girl in the Curl surf shop in Dana Point says, "Long-armed spring suits are cool because you don't get any tan lines."

＊**tip**

Most surfing wetsuits do up at the back, unlike diving and waterskiing wetsuits. Sure, this makes them trickier to do up, but the zip's there to make it more comfortable when you're lying on your board. You can always ask a cute guy on the beach to help do you up . . .

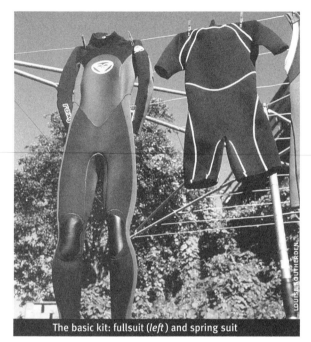

The basic kit: fullsuit (*left*) and spring suit

● Wetsuit jackets: long-sleeved neoprene tops that you wear with your boardshorts or bikini bottom. Great for chilly summer days.

Although wetsuits are getting more expensive, they're now softer, more flexible, more comfortable, warmer, and lighter than ever. They also last longer because they're better made, and there's now a huge range of girls' wetsuits, which wasn't always the case. The first fullsuit I ever bought was hot pink with bright blue arms and legs; it was the only one in the last surf shop I tried (none of the other shops even *had* girls' wetsuits), and I desperately wanted to keep surfing through winter so I wouldn't lose the skills I'd managed to pick up over the summer.

The trick to getting a wetsuit you'll get the most wear out of is choosing one that fits you and suits the area you'll be surfing. Ask around, see what other surfers are wearing, and ask your local surf shop what they recommend. If it's really cold, you might even need other accessories such as a wetsuit hood, gloves, or booties.

Every wetsuit is a trade-off between thickness and flexibility: It has to be thick enough to keep you warm but not so thick that you can't move your arms to paddle. Try on as many brands as you can, because they're all designed with different shapes in mind. The most important thing is that it fits snugly all over—you don't want any baggy bits where water's going to slosh around—while still allowing you to move freely. Paddling is the most strenuous thing you're going to be doing in the water, and you don't want to feel like you're pulling against a rubber band every time you reach forward. Make sure the suit's not too restrictive by doing a few full arm rotations; swing your arms about like a mad thing.

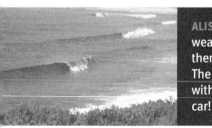

ALISON: If you're surfing somewhere really cold and you have to wear a hood, you may as well put conditioner in your hair and then put on a rubber swim cap and give yourself a hair treatment. The trouble is, I'm very tall and I'm quite strong, so in a wetsuit with a hood and gloves, I look like I'm about to break into your car!

Don't be afraid to move around in it, go for a stroll around the shop (make sure you smile at the other customers!). It might feel fine when you're standing there but pinch and sag in all the wrong places when you're lying down, standing up on your board, or twisting around to catch a wave. It's also a good idea to try on the wetsuit with a rash guard, if you're planning to wear one underneath, or with your bikini, to make sure the whole ensemble is going to be comfortable.

What else do you need?

Leashes

A leash (also called a legrope) is basically a length of stretchy polyurethane cord with a Velcro ankle strap at one end and a smaller strap that attaches to your board at the other. Your leash needs to be at least as long as your board. Since your board is going to be about 7 to 8 feet long, try to get a leash about 8 feet long, which will cost about $35. Most leashes have key pockets—great for keeping your car key safe, particularly when surfing at city beaches that are notorious for car thefts and break-ins.

In the early days of surfing, no self-respecting surfer would have been seen dead with a leash. Those were the days when men were men and boards, mostly longboards, were often damaged. When leashes were invented in the early 1970s, they were a huge breakthrough, not just for the safety and convenience of keeping a surfer close to her board, but because they allowed surfers to surf previously impossible breaks: beaches with rocky shorelines and, more significantly, reefs with perfect mechanically breaking waves.

These days, there are times when it's fun to surf without a leash, such as when it's almost flat and the chances of having to swim for your board are minimal, or when you're training yourself to have more board control and want a bit of exercise every time you lose your board.

But when you're just starting out, a leash is a must-have. Basically it keeps you and your board together (how romantic!). This means that whenever you lose contact with your board, all you have to do to get going again is reel it back to you and climb on. You won't have to swim whenever you wipe out or ditch your board. Your board won't endanger other surfers or swimmers when you fall off and it keeps going. And although you should never rely on your board completely for getting back to shore safely, it's comforting to know that with a leash, you have less chance of being separated from each other.

WET AND WARM

Is it true that surfers pee in their wetsuits? You bet. It might sound disgusting, but it's one of the best ways to warm up on a cold day! So relax and go with the flow. If it's any comfort, everyone else out there is probably doing it too and it's no different from peeing while you're swimming in the ocean—everything gets flushed out soon enough. Of course, if you're feeling shark-conscious (for example, when you're surfing at dusk or near a river mouth), it might be a good idea to hold on until you come in. And always rinse your wetsuit with freshwater after your surf!

✳tip

To stop wax from getting all over everything in your beach bag or the inside of your car, especially on hot summer days, keep it in a plastic bag or old soap container.

Of course, like any piece of equipment, leashes have their drawbacks: They can cause your board to spring back and hit you; they can get snagged on submerged rocks; they can tangle with other surfers when you wipe out too close to one another; or, as happened to me once, they can loop around your neck when you're still underwater (pretty scary). But their advantages far outweigh these disadvantages. Make sure you use one.

Wax

The least expensive but most essential item in your surfing kit is surf wax. It comes in all shapes and flavors, so choosing which kind to get is partly a matter of personal preference—when your nose is just inches from the deck of your board, do you want the scent of vanilla, coconut oil, root beer, or plumeria in your nostrils? And waxes come with the kinds of names only surfers could (or would) invent: Sex Wax, Sticky Bumps, Five Daughters, there's even surf wax for girls called Chicky Wax.

There are basically two kinds of wax: warm-water and cold-water wax. As the name suggests, warm-water wax is for summer and surf trips to tropical places. It doesn't melt as easily as cold-water wax, which is softer so you can apply it when the temperature outside is chilly. And there are waxes in between—if you're not sure which one to use for the place you'll be surfing, ask your local surf shop.

Wax goes on the deck of your board (the side you stand on) to stop your feet from slipping. Never wax the underside of your board—wax will slow it down and it won't be able to glide through the water.

A wax comb is also handy. This is a piece of plastic with a jagged edge on one side (for roughing up your wax when it gets too smooth and slippery) and a bladelike edge on the other (for removing wax from your board).

Wax vs. deck grip

An alternative to wax, deck grip is basically an adhesive piece of plastic with a grippy surface that you stick to the part of your board where you want the most traction. When starting out, you're better off using wax, simply because your board is going to be quite big and a complete set of deck grip will be pricey.

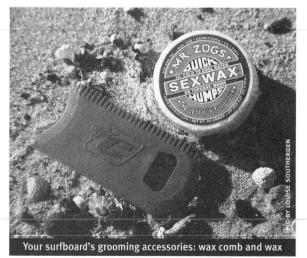

PIC BY LOUISE SOUTHERDEN

Your surfboard's grooming accessories: wax comb and wax

There are other advantages to wax. You can put wax right where you need it—and that might change as your surfing progresses: all over the board at first, then just where your feet go, and maybe where your hands grip the board when you duck-dive. Waxing your board can give you time to check the conditions before dashing headlong into the water; it's also a good warm-up for your arms. Borrowing wax is a great way to meet other surfers. It smells nice! And it's cheap—a bar of wax usually costs around $1.00 and will last for weeks (depending on how often you surf), whereas a tail pad (the cheapest deck grip you can buy) costs around $30.

Deck grip, on the other hand, can be great in hot climates, it doesn't get on your clothes when you're carrying your board, and you don't have to "wax up" before every surf—just grab your board and be the first in the water! And, as your surfing progresses, a tail pad (deck grip that you stick onto the tail of your board) can help you to place your back foot in the right spot every time. You can even use deck grip to brighten up your board. Some brands, like Island Style, have tail pads in cute shapes—dolphins, butterflies, hibiscus flowers—and pretty colors. The main disadvantages of grip are that it can get expensive, particularly if you want to change boards often, and it can also lose its stickiness and start to peel off after lots of exposure to the elements.

Surfboard bags

Do you need a bag or cover for your surfboard? It depends on how much traveling your board is going to do. If you're just taking it from house to car to beach, probably not. But if you want to go on weekend surf trips, take public transport to the beach, or strap your board to the roof of your car for a long trip, board bags can be very handy.

There are two kinds of surfboard bags. There are soft cloth covers to keep your board out of the sun (UV exposure makes white surfboards go yellow after a while) and protect it from minor bumps as you're transporting it to and from the beach. You can pick up a soft cover for about $40 from your local surf shop—or make one yourself.

A travel cover is a more serious affair. Made of toughened nylon, with a zipper that often runs the whole length of the board for ease of packing, and a strap you can sling over your shoulder, travel covers offer much more protection for your board. Some have hard plastic inserts to make them even tougher. They're also roomy enough to fit all your surfing gear—towels, wetsuits, bikinis, boardshorts, spare fins—which is great when

✳tip

Make sure you put your surfboard into its cover the same way every time. Otherwise, wax can end up on the bottom of your board. You can even write a W inside the cover on the wax side to remind yourself which way to put your board in.

*tip

To get zinc off your face at the end of a summer's day, use an exfoliant or facial scrub—it's gentler on your skin than tissues or a crusty old towel. And don't forget to moisturize afterward.

you're traveling; all you need to carry is a board bag and a day pack. You can get single, double, and even triple board bags (the last are eerily called "coffin bags" because they look so boxy). They start at around $100.

Sun protection

Gone are the days when surfers would go out for hours on end without so much as a smear of sunscreen across their noses. In one sense, we're lucky to be surfing in an era where we're more aware of the long-term damage of getting too many UV rays. The range of sunscreens available these days is mind-boggling, so you're sure to find one that suits your skin type and needs.

Personally, I always look for sunscreen that won't sting my eyes, stays on after a few hours in the water, and has an SPF of at least 30. Zinc oxide is excellent because it acts as a physical block instead of a chemical one, so it seems more effective for long exposure to the sun. A lot of the pro surfers wear zinc all over their faces, particularly when they're on surf trips in the tropics, for maximum sun protection. (More about sunscreen in Chapter 5.)

More and more surfers these days are wearing hats in the surf (to keep the sun off their faces) and even surf goggles (to reduce the glare). The latter are pretty expensive; a cheaper option is to tie a string around an old pair of sunglasses and wear them out in the water (it works!). Both are great for surf trips in tropical places, but generally not necessary for your daily session at your local beach.

Other stuff

Nose guards

Not for you, for your board! A nose guard is a rubber tip that fits over the nose of your surfboard to stop it from injuring you or someone else. They're not so important for longboards, which have rounded noses and are less likely to take out your eye, but they're essential for most shortboards. If you're riding a board with a pointy nose, get a nose guard from your local surf shop (they're about $12.95) and stick it on before you go for your first surf. They usually have self-adhesive tape inside them, so there's no need for messy glue. And if you notice that one of your friends' surfboards doesn't have one, buy her one

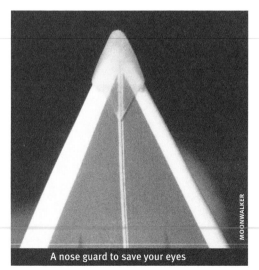
MOONWALKER
A nose guard to save your eyes

as a present; it shows you care (and might even save your own eyes if you surf together a lot).

Booties

There are two reasons to wear wetsuit booties: for the cold and for protection from rocks, coral reefs, sea urchins, and other prickly creatures. You can wear the same booties for both reasons, since they all have firm soles to prevent bits of reef and sea urchin spines from penetrating your soft soles, but you can get cold-weather booties with thicker neoprene for added warmth.

If you're surfing in Hawaii, Florida, or Southern California most of the time, you probably won't have much need for booties for warmth, even in winter. In Northern California or on the East Coast in winter, though, it's a different story. Make sure you get the ones that look like ankle boots; they'll stay on better than ones that are cut lower, though they all have adjustable Velcro straps.

If you're mostly surfing beach breaks, you won't need booties to protect your feet—even if you occasionally jump off the rocks to get into the water. The time to buy them is before you go on a tropical surf trip, where reef cuts can turn nasty in a fairly short time. They cost around $35.

Helmets

The main reasons to get a surf helmet are to protect your head in the event of a wipeout when you're surfing over reefs and rocks, and to protect your ears when you're surfing in cold water (too much exposure to cold water can cause a common complaint called "surfers' ear"). Some longboarders (those who ride 9-foot-plus boards) wear them to avoid concussion in the event that they hit their own board. Helmets can also save you from nasty fin chops to the side of the head.

That said, you probably won't need a surf helmet for some time. Even if you're worried about your board hitting you in the head, the cost (Gath helmets start at about $120) and inconvenience (they take some getting used to because they mess with your sense of balance) may outweigh the safety advantages. You're better off learning a few tricks to prevent the old "board in the head" syndrome, such as wrapping your arms over your head whenever you surface after a wipeout, and trying to be aware of where your board is at all times, even when you're underwater. Save the helmet-buying experience for further down the track, perhaps before your first big surf trip to Hawaii.

Ding repair kits

Repair kits are something that you usually don't buy until you ding your board, but it can be handy to keep a tube of Solarez in your car (small tubes cost about $9.95) if you don't live near any surf shops or if you're away on a surf trip.

Solarez (another brand is Ding All Suncure Resin) is a fast-curing easy-to-apply ding repair kit in a tube that's great for spontaneous repairs. All you need do to fix a ding is sandpaper it, squeeze some resin into it, put your board in the sun to harden the Solarez, and then sand it smooth. There's a huge range of repair kits now, including ones for bodyboard fins, wetsuits, and epoxy surfboards.

You can also buy resin, fiberglass matting, and small plastic bottles of catalyst, which you mix together for dings that require a bit more handiwork. Don't be fooled, though, ding repairing is an art, and when you're starting out it's a good idea to ask someone else (a friend or the surf shop where you bought your board) to fix your dings for you or at least show you how to do it. If you take your injured board to a surf shop, ding repairs cost from $20 for the most basic, up to about $100 to repair a snapped board.

Roof racks or soft racks?

You'll need racks if you're planning on transporting your board to the beach by car, assuming your board doesn't fit inside. Roof racks attach to your car's door rims. Soft racks are a cheaper option (around $30)—they're basically a set of straps with padded sleeves that allow you to tie boards to the roof of your car when you don't have fitted roof racks. Roof racks are better for long distances, but soft racks do the job for shorter home-to-beach trips.

BEL:
Go surfing with friends—because it's so intimidating as a girl to go out there by yourself. If you have another girl with you, you can laugh. It's so much easier to laugh at yourself when there's someone else there.

A few other essentials

A dash of confidence. It's a little-known fact that confidence often comes before ability. Sure, if you can do something well, it's easy to be confident. The trick is to be confident that you *will* be able to surf, sooner or later—which is actually more about trust than confidence. It's about trusting that if you put your time in, get out there as often as you can, pay attention, and give it all you've got, you'll get where you want to go.

Patience. There are going to be days when you go for a surf and don't catch a single wave. Or when you catch only one wave out of every ten you go for. Or when every wave you do catch ends in a decidedly ungraceful dismount, probably in front of that cute surfer boy you've been trying to impress all morning. Later on, when your surfing progresses, you'll need patience to wait for waves, to watch other surfers riding waves without wishing it were you, and to wait for swells.

A sense of humor. No one ever said you were going to look good while you learn to surf! And whether you're springing to your feet while your board is still on the sand, wiping out in ways that have never been tried before, or botching a takeoff on a two-foot wave, it helps to be able to laugh at yourself and not take it (or yourself) too seriously. Remember why you're here: to have fun. The trick is to keep your expectations low and try to enjoy every step of the weird and wonderful process of learning to surf.

Time. You need time to get used to the feel of your board before you even think about standing up. Surfing only one or two days a week may not be enough at first, because by the time you've got used to surfing again, it's time to give it up for another week.

Friends to surf with. If you surf with friends who are at the same level as you, you'll feel less self-conscious and have more fun!

A go-for-it attitude. Surfing has to be fun, but you'll progress faster if you have a certain amount of dedication, too. Try going out when the waves are mushy or the wind's onshore, even when you don't feel like it. Try having no expectations and see how it feels. Set little goals for yourself, like catching three waves this session, or standing up on every wave, or trying to turn.

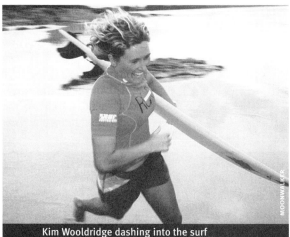

Kim Wooldridge dashing into the surf

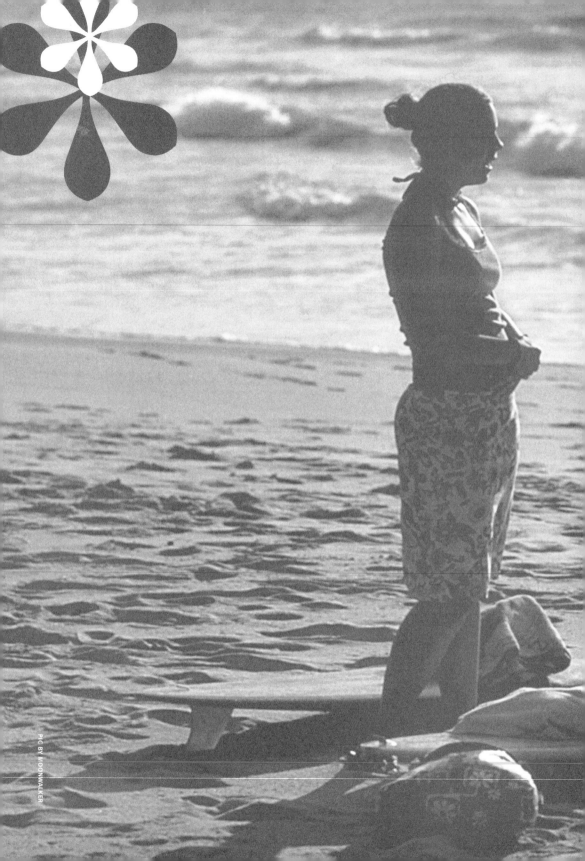

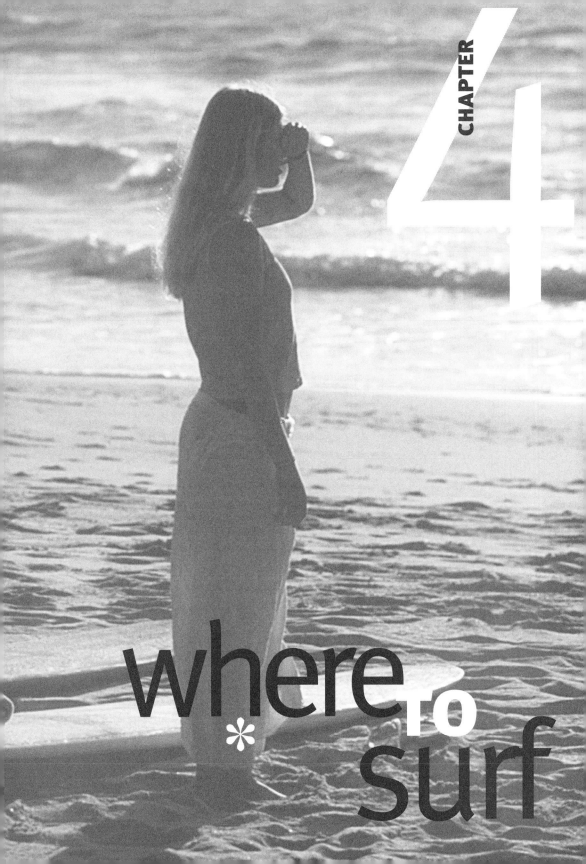

where *to surf

Learn:

Why surfers need to understand the weather. **About different types of waves and how they're formed.** How waves are affected by wind, tide, sandbanks, and the shape of the coast. **What kinds of waves are good for first-timers.** The when and where of wave prediction. **How to check the swell: using surf report websites, weather maps.** The art of the surf check—what to look for when you're checking the surf. **How to measure wave size.**

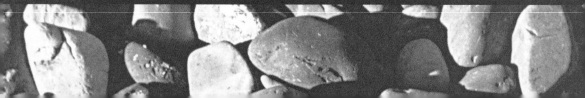

A s you've probably gathered by now, there's more to surfing than just being able to stand up on a surfboard. In the words of a longtime surfer I once met, "Surfers don't ride surfboards, they ride waves." And to ride waves you have to understand them, even just a little. You also have to know where to find them.

What's the weather got to do with it?

Nonsurfers are often mystified by the things surfers see when they gaze out at the ocean. It's as if the waves are in the eye of the beholder; if you can't surf, you probably can't see them. But as soon as you start thinking about surfing, your whole perspective begins to shift. You start noticing how the waves are breaking, whether there's any wind, where other surfers are paddling out. . . . It's amazing what you see when you start looking at the ocean from the point of view of getting out there and riding its waves— it's almost as if you never really saw it before.

Behind this new perspective, however, there's something else. Hang around surfers long enough, and you'll soon notice that when they're not talking about surfing and waves they're talking about the weather. There's a good reason for this: no surf spot on Earth gets good waves every day. Which means that if you understand a bit about the weather and the way different conditions create and affect waves, you're more likely to find good waves more often.

Why not just wait for the waves to come? That's definitely an option: check your local beach every morning, surf if there are waves, and do something else if there aren't. Lots of surfers live like this, particularly if they don't have a car to check nearby beaches, and it does keep life simple.

The advantage of understanding the weather and how it affects the surfing environment, however, is that you get to surf more.

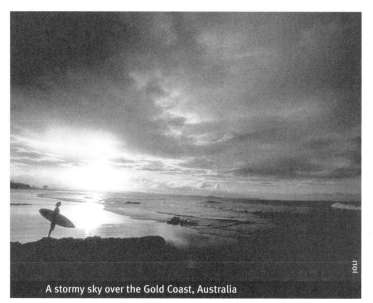

A stormy sky over the Gold Coast, Australia

So instead of giving up on surfing to go to the movies with your friends when the waves are no good at your local beach, you know to check the beach around the corner, because it faces a different direction and therefore might have good waves (unless you *really* want to go to the movies). Or if the waves aren't so good now, but you know that your local beach is often better at a lower tide, you can still go do something else, knowing that you can probably get a surf later.

If you take this weather know-how a step further by learning how to read weather maps and use surf report websites and other sources, you can even anticipate when there might be waves and plan ahead. Then there's the joy of the search: understanding the weather helps you find waves when you're traveling up or down the coast or even overseas, since the same principles pretty much apply worldwide.

Even if all this weren't true, trying to learn to surf without learning something about the weather is virtually impossible: just sitting on the beach and watching the ocean, you can't help but learn about the wind, waves, and tides. Plus, you've got an incentive to learn: to surf perfect waves. So take in as much or as little as you like, watch, listen, check the surf as often as you can, and try to notice subtle changes.

Following is a bit of theory to get you started. It might look like a lot to absorb, but it's nothing compared to what you'll learn just by going out in the water and being aware of your surroundings. And you don't have to learn it all before you learn to surf; you can always come back to it later if you're not sure why the wind messed up the waves or why the surf was great at high tide but lousy at low tide.

Wind + water = waves

If you only remember one thing about weather and waves, make sure it's this: Waves are created by wind. Try blowing across the surface of a swimming pool or pond, or even a glass of water, and you'll see for yourself that when air moves over water it creates ripples. Now imagine this effect on a larger scale: that is, the wind blowing across the ocean.

There are basically two kinds of waves, both created by wind.

Wind swell. If the wind has been blowing steadily toward the beach all day, you can pretty much stake your life on the fact that there'll be at least a few waves by late afternoon. Waves created by local winds like this are called "wind swell," and they tend to be close together (that is, one wave breaks and then another one breaks right behind it) and even a bit bumpy, but they're perfectly rideable, particularly when the wind dies, leaving the surface of the ocean smooth and glassy.

Ground swell. These waves are created by stronger winds farther off the coast, usually from a low pressure system, blowing across a greater distance, or "fetch." You can recognize ground swell by one main feature: The waves come in groups called "sets," with long lulls in between. Surfers love ground swell for several reasons: the waves have more power than wind swell, which makes them more exciting and challenging to ride; the lulls between sets make it easier to paddle out; and the waves arrive in more neatly arranged corduroy lines, which, when they hit certain surf spots, create those dream waves you see in surfing magazines.

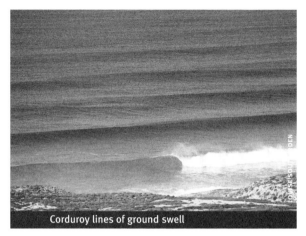
Corduroy lines of ground swell

Types of waves

You've probably heard surfers say no two waves are exactly the same. But even waves, being natural entities, behave according to a few rules. Generally speaking, for a wave to break, the water underneath it has to be shallower than the wave's height. So when you see waves breaking, you can get some idea of the depth of the water. Small waves need less water under them to break, while big waves can break in fairly deep water (a comforting thought when you're preparing to launch yourself into one!).

In surfspeak, a "surf break" is literally where waves break. There are three kinds of surf breaks, which translates to three places where you can (theoretically) find waves:

- **Beach breaks:** where the waves break over sand, with access usually from a sandy beach. These are great for learning to surf, plus there's often a choice of spots to surf along the beach (known as "peaks"), so you might be able to find one that's uncrowded. Just remember, though: not all beach breaks are beginner-friendly. Some of the heaviest waves in the world break over sand, and it's not all soft landings: A solid beach break can snap boards (or cause injury) as easily as any reef if the waves are powerful enough.

● **Point breaks:** where the waves wrap around a headland or a point. As long as the waves aren't too big and they break over sand, point breaks are ideal for learning to surf, for several reasons. Paddling out is a dream, because you don't have to get through whitewater; you can just paddle wide of the breaking waves, where it's deep. You're less likely to run into other surfers than you are at a beach break, where people are paddling out through the break. And the waves tend to peel along the point in one direction, so the rides are longer and you have a chance to really get a feel for having a surfboard under your feet.

● **Reef breaks:** where the waves break over a hard surface, usually rock, coral, or something man-made (there are artificial surfing reefs made of old truck tires and sand-filled bags). Because you're surfing over a hard surface, which increases the risk of serious injury if you wipe out, reef breaks tend to be for experienced surfers. However, small waves on reef breaks can be great for honing your skills because every wave breaks mechanically along the edge of the reef, giving you a chance to focus on your surfing instead of the waves' unpredictability. Most of the best surfing spots in the world are reef breaks, such as those in Hawaii, Puerto Rico, Costa Rica, Indonesia, Fiji, the Maldives, Tahiti, and Tonga.

Conditions to look for

Just to complicate matters, there's more to finding surf than looking for waves. The next step is to recognize the conditions that affect the waves, most importantly the Big Four: tide, wind, sandbanks, and the shape of the coast.

✳tip

Keep a tide chart (available free at most West Coast surf shops) in the glove compartment of your car or in your surf bag—it's handy to check what the tide's doing when you get to the beach.

The tide. Tides affect how waves break by changing the depth of the water, often by several feet. There are usually two high tides and two low tides every day, generally about six hours apart. Tide times vary by about an hour every day: for example, if high tide today was at 4:05 A.M., tomorrow it's at 5:05 A.M. The amount of water moving in and out with the tide changes daily too, depending on the phase of the moon; the difference between high and low tide is usually greatest around a full moon and a new moon, which can make for dramatic changes in the surf.

What this means: Every surf spot works on different tides, but there are a few guidelines. Often the best time to surf is about halfway between low tide and high tide, on an incoming tide: that is, about two to three hours after low tide. High tide tends to make waves slower, there's less whitewater to ride, and there can be a lot of water moving around; low tide tends to make waves faster and more hollow so takeoffs are more critical. At very low tide, waves can just close out.

Wind direction. Generally speaking, "offshore" winds, blowing off the land toward the sea, make the waves better for surfing than "onshore" winds, blowing from the sea to the beach. To determine where the wind's coming from, look at the surface of the ocean (not the waves, but the surface of the waves); offshore winds make the waves look smooth, onshore winds make the waves look choppy and messy.

What this means: Surfers love offshore breezes because they smooth the surface of the ocean, making the waves easier to ride; onshore winds make the waves crumble and break earlier than they otherwise would, making for lots of closeouts. In terms of generating waves, however, onshore winds are better because they push waves into the beach; offshore winds, if they blow hard enough and long enough, can flatten the ocean into something resembling a lake. But basically the rule is: offshore good, onshore bad.

Sandbars or sandbanks, and reefs. When surfers talk about banks they're not discussing their finances; they're talking about mounds or banks of sand—under the waves. Why? Because these sandbars—which shift constantly in response to big swells and storms—determine whether your local beach break will be good for surfing.

What this means: If the banks are no good, the waves won't be either, no matter what the swell, wind, and tide are doing. At reef breaks, however, the bottom contours are virtually constant, so determining whether the waves will be good on any one day is a much simpler process: all you have to take into account are the tide and the wind and swell direction. Some reefs, for example, only break when there's a south swell, a northeast wind, and a rising tide; it might seem limiting but being so reliable allows surfers in the know to predict the best time to surf there.

Coastal curves. The direction a beach faces will determine how it reacts to certain swell and wind directions. When you get to know the way the coastline curves in your area, you'll discover that each beach faces the ocean at a slightly different angle. Where I live, on Sydney's northern beaches, there are more than twenty beaches, facing almost every conceivable direction. Also, the more convoluted the coastline, the more choices you'll have about where to surf.

What this means: When you know your coastline and you

> **THE ANSWER IS BLOWING IN THE WIND . . .**
> Experienced surfers can often tell which way the wind's blowing just by its smell. An onshore wind smells salty because it's coming off the sea. Offshore winds, like California's dry Santa Ana winds that blow off the desert, have a more earthy smell. The temperature of the wind can give it away too: an onshore wind is usually cool; offshore winds vary depending on the season (cool in winter, warm in summer).

know where the wind and swell are coming from that day, you have a better chance of scoring good waves.

Where should I surf?

The first few times you go surfing, you probably won't need to ask yourself this question because you'll either have no choice about where you surf (if there're waves you'll go, and if it's too rough you won't) or you'll be with someone (like a surfing instructor) who can point out where to surf safely. It's also not going to make too much difference where you surf at first—you basically just want a beach, preferably with a sandy bottom, with lines of gentle whitewater rolling in.

As you get more confident and independent, however, you'll probably want to explore more and more beaches, and that's when it helps to know what kinds of waves to look for. The two most important things to remember are to stay safe and have fun— which is easier said than done, I know, when you're feeling like a small drowned creature attached to a large unwieldy surfboard, but it's all about the process!

Basically, you want to slow things down a bit. There's enough to learn about handling a surfboard and managing your own skills without throwing yourself in the deep end as far as waves go.

First things first: Head for the whitewater

Starting in the whitewater helps you get a feel for riding the waves without having to stare down a sheer wall of green that threatens to pitch you end over end (who said surfing isn't fun?). (Chapter 7 covers this in more detail.)

Ready for the real thing?

When you're ready to try some unbroken green waves, make sure they are:

- Small: no bigger than waist high when you're standing on your board.
- Full: more like a gentle ramp than a halfpipe.
- Breaking in plenty of water: if it's too shallow, the waves will break too quickly and you'll probably start to worry (with good reason!) that you could hit your head on the bottom when you fall off your board.
- Breaking over sand: that is, a classic beach break. Compared to surfing over rocks or coral reef, surfing over sand is safer,

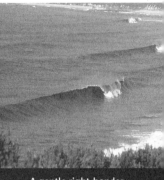

KATE SKARRATT, PRO SURFER AND SURF COACH: The best thing to do when you're learning is to sit and assess the conditions before you go out. Ask the lifeguard or other surfers around, don't go straight out to the spot that's most packed with the most people: you'll have more fun if you can find a peak with just a few people and a nice gentle wave. Don't wear yourself out in waves that are dumping, because it can really get you down—you'll end up being exhausted and not catching anything. If you can find a bank that's got nice little lefts and rights or a point break that's really small and gentle—they're the waves you'll have more fun on.

A gentle right-hander

less threatening (you can catch the whitewater straight in to the beach when you want to come in), and generally easier, since you don't have to worry about hitting the bottom (if you do, sand is generally more forgiving than rock).

● Breaking gently (peeling) along their length: You have time to stand up, get your balance, and maybe even ride along the wave a little.

● Breaking, full stop: Before you paddle out, check for whitewater; that's a good indication that the waves out there are breaking. If the waves aren't breaking, you can always get out there anyway and practice your paddling.

● Uncrowded: When it comes to finding a good surf spot for learning, less of a crowd means more surfing practice. Although learning how to surf safely with others is an intrinsic part of surfing, you've got the rest of your surfing life to learn those skills. For now, look for beaches with plenty of space. It's easier to relax and pay attention to what you're doing when you're not thinking about bumping into other surfers or swimmers or feeling self-conscious about spectators.

Knowing your rights from your lefts

When waves break, the whitewater moves along the face of the wave, either to the right or the left. (Some waves break simultaneously along their entire length, making them virtually unrideable; they're called "closeouts"). That's why surfers describe waves as right-handers ("rights") and left-handers ("lefts"). Which is which? The direction a wave breaks is from the *surfer's* viewpoint as she's looking back at the beach. So a right-hander is a wave that breaks to the right as you're looking back at the beach or riding it. From the beach, therefore, a right-hander breaks to the left. A left-hander breaks to the left as you're riding it.

Finding waves—the when and where of wave prediction

In theory, you can find surfable waves anywhere there's an ocean and the right configuration of coastline, as long as you know just two things: when and where to look. The "when" means finding out if there's any swell and if the swell's getting bigger (picking up) or smaller (dropping), checking the tide times, and knowing when the wind is coming up. The "where" means knowing your local coastline like the back of your hand: knowing which beaches receive swell from a certain direction, which beaches are good in certain winds, and whether they work on low or high tides.

To show how they go together, here's a short surf story. It's summer and you've got tomorrow off to go surfing. Great! You could just get up when you wake up, throw your board in the car, and head to the beach. But to maximize your water time (and minimize your driving-around-checking-the-surf time), it's a good idea to start planning now:

● Go to bed early so you can get up early, preferably at dawn. Because it's summer, the sea breeze is probably going to come in and mess up the surf by midmorning, if not earlier. The sooner you get out there, the less crowded it will be, and the waves are more likely to be glassy and easier to surf. The sun's not as brutal as later in the day, too. It's just more pleasant all-round. The rule is: surf early, unless the tide tells you otherwise.

● So what are the tides doing? Check your local newspaper for tomorrow's high and low tide times (if it doesn't list tomorrow's tides, find out today's times and add an hour). Let's say high tide is at 9 A.M. At most beach breaks, high tide isn't the best time to surf, which means you'll want to get in the water at least a couple of hours before nine. So far, you've got the "when" sorted. Now for the "where."

● Is there any swell about right now? Check the weather map in today's paper or watch tonight's TV weather forecast. Even if they don't mention swell, you can still gather lots of info, such as wind direction and temperature (even water temperature). Better still, call one of your friends who went surfing today. If she tells you there's a smallish north swell (a swell that's coming from the north), you know that your local beach—

DAWN PATROL

Ever wondered why dedicated surfers get up so early? It's because the wind tends to be offshore or nonexistent in the morning, thanks to the heating and cooling of the land relative to the sea. It works like this: The land heats up and cools down much more than the sea, which tends to hold its temperature. Because warm air rises, it attracts more air toward it to take its place. In the early mornings, particularly in summer, the sea is warmer than the land so air moves from land to sea—that is, offshore. When the sun begins to warm up the land, the air moves back again, creating an onshore sea breeze. The reverse often happens in the late afternoon, so you get offshore breezes again. In winter, you can often get offshore winds all day because the sea-breeze phenomenon isn't as strong as the effect of weather systems such as low pressures over the coast.

let's call it Shaggies—isn't going to be getting any waves because it faces south and is protected from north swells. A better spot would be Nobodys, a nice beach across the bay from Shaggies that is open to north swells and will still be good before high tide at nine.

● How about the wind? The TV forecast predicts a southwest wind (a typical summer sea breeze on the West Coast). That's good news, because everybody knows Nobodys is protected from southwest winds.

So now you know you can go straight to Nobodys tomorrow morning. If it's no good, you can always check somewhere else, but at least you didn't waste time at Shaggies.

Checking the swell

Although there are lots of factors that affect waves, the thing that impacts most on surfers' lives is swell: that is, whether or not there are waves. Even if the wind, tide, and sandbars are all perfect, if there's no swell, you can't surf. (Of course, the opposite can also be true: Sometimes there's swell, but the wind, tide, and sandbars at your local beach are all wrong, but at least you've got more chance of finding somewhere surfable.) This is why surfers are constantly surf-obsessed.

How do you check the swell? At its simplest, checking the swell means heading down to your local beach, where you'll be able to see if there are waves or not. But what happens if you can't get to the beach or your local beach, like Shaggies, above, is protected from the prevailing swell?

Thankfully, there are now more "surf check shortcuts"—ways

to check the swell without being at the beach—than ever before. The two most reliable resources surfers use are surf report websites and weather maps.

Surf report websites

The best thing about surf websites is that they're designed by surfers for surfers, so all the relevant information is at your fingertips: tide times, swell size, often live photos of the surf (surf cams), wind direction, swell direction, even water temperature. Here are a few to get you started:

● **Wetsand** (www.wetsand.com/wavecast). A great user-friendly site with surf reports and swell forecasts for California (Northern, Central, and Southern), the East Coast (northern, southern, and Gulf of Mexico), and Costa Rica. You can also get surf reports for Baja, Hawaii, Central America, Peru, Tobago, Fiji, Indonesia, and Tonga. You can even sign up to receive free surf reports by e-mail.

● **Surfersvillage surf forecast** (www.surforecast.com). This is a good site for an overview of the conditions in your area. Color-coded maps show wave height and direction, tides, sea surface temperatures, wind speed and direction, and satellite photos, as well as surf cams for specific beaches and links to buoy data.

● **Surfline** (www.surfline.com). Surf reports are just one of the offerings on this magazine-style site—there's even a cool Women's Channel. But back to the surf reports: click on "cams and reports" to watch real-time video footage of the waves at your local surf spot right now and a description of the conditions including wind, waves, and tide times. You can also access Surfline.com reports from your cell phone or subscribe to a more-detailed premium surf forecast service.

● **Buoyweather** (www.buoyweather.com). Although parts of this site are accessible to subscribers only, there are some great free forecasts showing wave height, swell direction, and wind strength and direction at six-hour intervals over the next five days. Go to Virtual Buoys, select your part of the world (say, North America) and zero in on a specific area (say, Florida). The data comes from instruments on buoys anchored to the sea floor at various locations around the world.

● **Stormsurf** (www.stormsurf.com). This San Francisco–based site specializes in big-wave surf forecasts for experienced surfers, but it does have surf meteorology tutorials for surfers of any level wanting to learn a bit about the ocean, as well as surf reports and surf forecasts for the Atlantic, Indian, and Pacific Ocean coasts.

There are loads more localized surf report sites too, like www.surfingsandiego.com in Southern California. To find a good surf report site in your area, check at your local surf shop or ask other surfers.

Weather maps

When you're just starting out, you probably won't need to decipher a weather map to predict swell; there are so many other sources for up-to-date wave information (see below). But as your surfing progresses, it can become a useful skill, particularly when you're on a surf trip where the only source of information is a local newspaper or TV weather report.

It's probably safe to say that most weather forecasters aren't surfers, so when they give the weather report, they're not going to tell you what the waves are like. Not in so many words, anyway. You have to read between the lines or, more accurately, read the lines on the weather map.

Reading a weather map is easy when you know what to look for, and when you're a surfer you want to find the lines called isobars that swirl over the ocean nearest to your local surf spot on the map. Isobars indicate air pressure and the movement of air (wind) around low and high pressure systems, signified by L and H on your map. When the lines are close together, that means the winds are strong (there's often a key with the map indicating how strong); when they're farther apart, it means lighter winds.

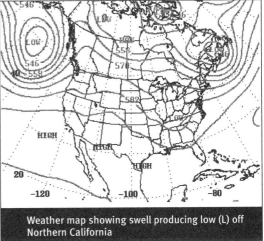

Weather map showing swell producing low (L) off Northern California

As for wind direction, the thing to remember is that in the northern hemisphere winds travel counterclockwise around low pressure systems and clockwise around high pressure systems (it's reversed in the southern hemisphere). So when you see closely spaced isobars around a low pressure system, you can work out the strength and direction of the wind and, because wind creates waves, you'll be able to get an idea of the expected size and direction of the swell. It won't tell you exactly when it's coming, but checking your local beach will tell you when it's arrived!

Other ways to check the surf without going to the beach

Most of us don't have the privilege of looking out our bedroom windows to a view of our local surf spot, but there are other ways to check the waves from home:

- **Read a newspaper.** In places where surfers make up a fair chunk of the population (such as Hawaii and parts of California), newspapers often give detailed surf reports on the weather page.

- **Call your local surf shop.** Even if it's not located right on the beach, the staff there will know what the surf is doing. They've probably even been surfing already, or if they haven't they might tell you why (it's flat, the waves are mushy or too big, the wind's all wrong).

- **Listen to the surf report on the radio.** If they don't mention your local beach, they'll give you some information (like wind direction, tide times, how big the swell is) that you can piece together to decide if your beach has any waves.

- **Dial-a-surf report.** These prerecorded surf reports that give water and air temperatures, tide times, wind direction and strength, and surfing conditions are just a phone call away. Check your local telephone directory under Surf Report. Some surf shops also have recorded messages detailing surfing conditions.

- For the ultimate in personalized surf checks, **call a friend who lives at the beach.** Or arrange for your friend to check the surf and then call you if the surf's worth getting out of bed for!

SAFETY FIRST, AND LAST

When you're checking the surf, make sure you think about not only how you're going to paddle out, but how you're going to come in. If your leash breaks or comes off and you lose your board, remember to swim in through the breaking waves, not the rip that carried you out there. If you're surfing at a patrolled beach where there are lifeguards on duty, be aware of any signs they may have stuck in the sand, warning of strong currents, submerged rocks, or other dangerous conditions. If you haven't surfed there before, you can even go and ask one of the lifeguards for tips. You never know, they might be surfers too.

● **Step outside.** This is a good one to do in your pj's early in the morning—you'd be surprised how much you can tell just by standing outside (unless you live more than twenty minutes from the beach, and then the conditions there might be pretty different from the conditions at your house). Is there any wind? Can you smell anything besides your brother's old sneakers on the back step? Maybe you can smell salt in the air (an indicator of a sea breeze—no good for surfing) or the warm, earthy smell of the land (an indicator of an offshore breeze—good for surfing).

The art of the surf check

Sooner or later, you're going to find yourself at the source: the beach itself. All the online surf reports and TV weather forecasts in the world are nothing compared to heading down to the beach and having a look at the waves for yourself. The trick is knowing what to look for and how to decode what you see in front of you.

A "surf check" list: what to look for when you get to the beach

● Is there any wind? If not, get out there! Glassy conditions can be lovely to surf in. If there is a breeze, how strong is it? Which way is it blowing? Is it onshore, offshore, or sideshore (blowing sideways across the beach)? You can check this on the way to the beach by looking at the way flags are flying. Otherwise, kick up some sand and see which way it falls. If the wind's strong enough and you have long hair, turn your head and see which way your hair blows.

● What's the tide doing? Is it coming in or going out? How close is it to low or high tide?

● What are the waves like? Are there clear peaks, or is it more like a washing machine out there? If you can't see any waves breaking, wait a few minutes—you might have arrived between sets (many a surfer has driven past her local beach in this lull time, concluded that it's flat, and driven home, only to find later that her buddies had a great surf).

● Are there any other surfers out? Where did they paddle out? Where are they

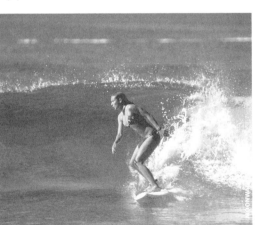
How big do you think this wave is?

sitting? Are they getting any waves, are they going right or left, are the rides long or short? If you see a surfer coming in, ask what it was like out there. Or ask another surfer checking the surf what she thinks the conditions are like, how the tide might affect them, and if she's going out or not.

If it looks good, it's time to go surfing! If you're not sure, spend a bit more time checking conditions. There's no rush and conditions change all the time, sometimes for the better, sometimes for the worse. The tide might drop, the currents might change, the wind might pick up, it might get more or less crowded. Watch and learn.

How big are the waves?

Ask a bunch of surfers that question, and their answers are likely to vary enormously. Most surfers look at the person riding the wave (or imagine someone riding it) and go from there, but even then it gets confusing. Why? Because the way waves are measured is one of the mysteries of surf culture.

Basically there are two schools of thought on this slippery matter. First, there are those who simply **measure the face of the wave**, which makes sense, because not only is that the part you see from the beach, it's the part you ride. So when you hear someone say it's "six foot" and you know they're talking wave faces (and assuming the average surfer is six feet tall) you know the waves are about head high. By this reckoning the wave in the photo (on page 95) is 5 to 6 foot.

Why would anyone do it any other way, you ask? Because waves break differently at different beaches, and the same size swell can manifest as different-sized waves. So the second way of talking about wave size is to **estimate the swell size**, the reasoning being that swell size is more meaningful than the face of a wave. The problem is that estimating swell size is a tricky thing. Most surfers will look at a breaking wave, see how high its face is, halve that figure, and give or take a foot (see?). So that 5-to-6-foot wave suddenly becomes 2 to 3 foot. Of course, if everyone speaks the same language, because they live in the same area and think about waves the same way, there's no confusion at all. There's also a little of that macho thing of underestimating wave size. That is, if you call a wave "6 foot" and it's really 12 foot, it makes you sound like a legend. Hawaiian surfers are notorious for this; if they see a wave with a 60-foot face, it's said to be "20-foot Hawaiian style."

There is a third option that's clearer and easier to understand than both of the above, no matter who you are, where you come from, or what surf language you speak: **measure the wave face**

using surfers as your point of reference. That is, you can say the waves are shoulder high, head high, overhead, double overhead, and, after that, huge! At least you won't come to blows with anyone about under- or over-estimating waves.

Last words

Be positive. Sometimes waves are better than they look from the beach. It might look messy and all over the place but you only need one or two good rides to make you feel that paddling out was worthwhile. Plus, less-than-classic conditions keep the crowds down so you might have the waves to yourself.

Surf as often as you can. Even when it's onshore, when the waves are small, when you don't feel like it. The trick is to get as many waves as you can when you're starting out. So go out for just twenty minutes or half an hour with no expectations; treat it as a practice session, and see how many waves you can catch in half an hour! To maximize your wave count, try sitting closer to the beach and catching the smaller waves that no one else is catching.

If it's completely flat, take your board out for a paddle. It'll keep your arm muscles strong and you'll get used to the feel of your board underneath you—so you'll be ready when the waves do come.

Be patient. Being a surfer means more than just being able to ride waves. It means understanding and respecting the ocean's cycles, as well as your own (the ones that make you a confident surfer one day and a kook the next). It means accepting the flat spells with grace and making the most of waves when they do come. There's a lot to be said for waiting out the flat spells with good humor, knowing it will all change soon enough.

Lower your expectations. I've had some of the best surfs when I didn't expect to (and some of the worst surfs when the waves were perfect!). It's all about what happens inside your head. When you don't have high expectations, you can end up having more fun than you thought you would. In any case, surfing usually makes you feel better than you did before you went out. Former world champion Pam Burridge once said that what attracted her to surfing was the freedom and the fact that "you came out of the water feeling better than when you went in, no matter how the surf was."

LOATA:
I improved heaps quicker because I went surfing in anything. If the waves are sucky, you learn to stand up really quickly. If they're taking their time, you learn to do a few more turns on each wave. You can't wait for the perfect wave, because it's so inconsistent. And even when it's flat, you can still go for a paddle to keep fit.

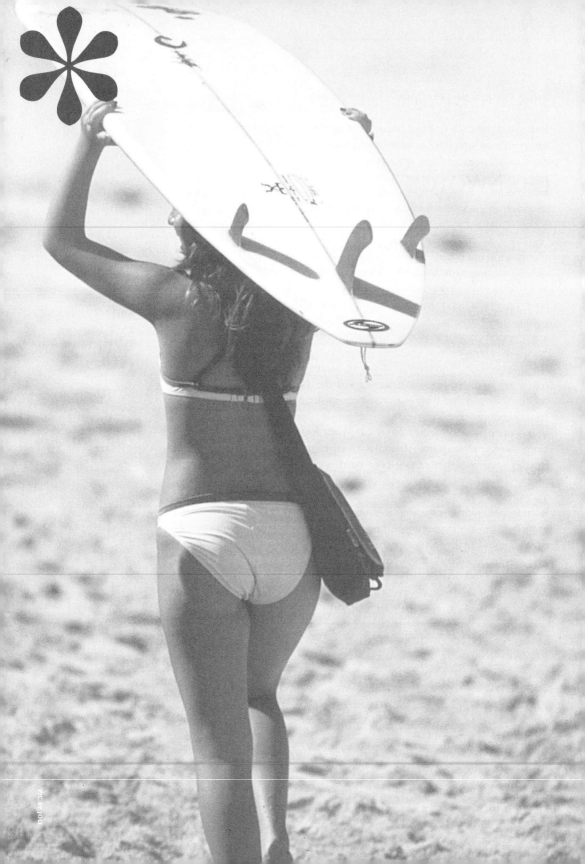

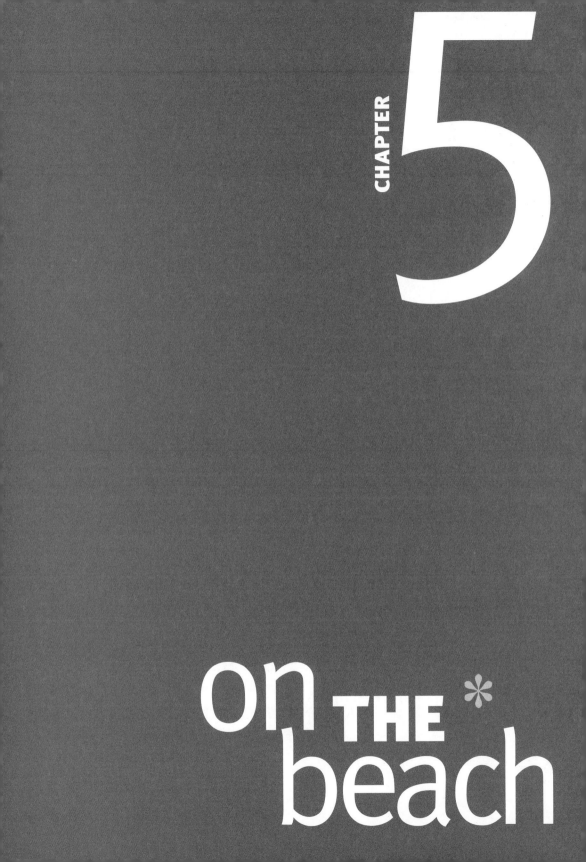

CHAPTER 5

on THE *
beach

Learn:

Tricks for getting changed easily on the beach. **How to wax your surfboard and attach your leash.** How to carry your board to the water's edge. **Stretches and yoga for surfing.** Which leg to put your leash on. **What to take to the beach.**

E very surfer has her own pre-surf ritual for getting ready—it might be the way she waxes her board, or whether she puts her bathing suit on in the parking lot or before she leaves home—and you'll find your own too. For now, however, here are a few tips for getting ready for your first surf.

Get your gear on

Ever wondered what possesses surfers to get into all sorts of strange contortions when changing into their wetsuits beside their car at the beach? Why do we put our bikini on when we get to the beach instead of just putting it on under our clothes before we leave home?

There's a simple explanation. Unless you're committed to going for a surf no matter what (and this is a fantastic attitude to have when you're starting out, because you need as much water time as you can get), you often need to see what the surfing conditions are like before you decide to go out. Sometimes you might check the surf several times a day, so putting on your swimsuit before you head down each time would be a pain. Plus, wearing street clothes to the beach ensures that you have something dry to put on after your surf: great after those marathon sessions when you're feeling slightly chilled.

There's no easy way to get changed at the beach, but it does get easier with practice. Skirts are great because you can slip your bikini on underneath with ease. So are tank tops (no sleeves to fuss with) and halter-neck bikinis. An old surfer's trick is to wrap your towel around you like a skirt and slip your bikini bottoms on underneath.

Winter changing rituals

Things definitely get a bit trickier in winter, with more layers and wetsuits to cope with, and colder fingers. Speed is your friend in the colder months: the aim is to minimize the time standing next to your car with the cold offshore wind threatening to whip your towel off your half-naked body. Or you can just get into your wetsuit at home—then drive home in your wetsuit after your surf and strip off under a hot shower (very reviving after a bone-chilling session).

If you do get changed at the beach, it's a good idea to get your board ready first (wax, leash, and so on), then get into your wetsuit to maximize time in the cocoon of your winter woolies. I have a friend who never wears anything under her wetsuit—she swears it's much more comfortable than wearing a bikini and a rash guard—and it probably is, but she has to be Harry Houdini when she's getting in and out of the darn thing (without giving the boys in the parking lot a peep show, that is).

SERENA BROOKE: I always take two bikinis to the beach—one to wear in the water and one to put on when I come in. It's good to have a pair of dry shorts to change into after your surf, too, particularly if you have to walk back from the beach. You can get a rash on your legs if you walk in wet boardshorts.

How to wax your board

If you've ever tried to lie on an unwaxed board, you'll know from bitter experience that wax is not a luxury item. It stops you from slipping off your surfboard, whether you're lying, sitting, or standing on it.

To wax your board, grab the bar of surf wax in one hand and rub it over the deck of your board in a circular motion (just like the Karate Kid: wax on, wax off). Keep waxing until small bumps appear—they're going to help you stay on your board.

Where to wax?

Basically, you need to apply wax everywhere you think your feet are going to go. Some longboarders wax right up to the nose of the board for nose riding, while experienced shortboarders often only wax two spots: where their front and back feet go. When you're starting out, it's a good idea to give yourself some leeway: wax the back two-thirds of the board. It's even a good idea to wax where your hands grab the board to duck-dive or turtle-roll under oncoming waves—if your board gets away from you in mid-duck dive/roll, it can head-butt you square in the face. Not pretty!

Just a reminder: wax the deck of your board, the side you stand on, not the bottom. Unlike skis or snowboards that need wax on the bottom to help them glide across the snow, surfboards glide through water just fine by themselves. In fact, waxing the bottom of your surfboard will slow it down and make it sluggish to ride. Try to keep the bottom of your board completely wax-free. Boards often pick up bits of wax from the inside of your board cover, from being in your car, or from your friends' boards, so check it now and then and pick off any stray bits before you hit the water. If you're stacking boards on top of one another, try to put their decks together or put a towel between them to stop wax from getting on the bottom of the boards.

How often should you wax your board?

You don't need to wax your board every time you surf, but you should check that it has enough wax before every surf. Just

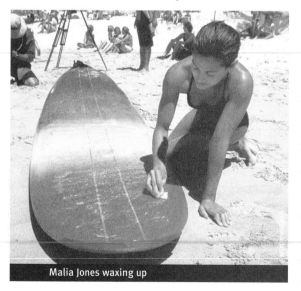

Malia Jones waxing up

rub your hand over the deck. If it feels "grippy," there's enough wax. If it feels smooth, you might want to put on more wax or rough up the wax that's already there with a wax comb. Drag the wax comb diagonally across your board, making sure the teeth go right into the wax to make clear lines; then drag it diagonally the other way so you make a crisscross pattern. This gives the wax that's already on your board more grip.

Wax on, wax off

One of the easiest ways to keep your surfboard shipshape is to strip the old wax off and apply a fresh coat. When wax has been on your board for too long, it starts to look pretty grimy: sand and bits of grass will stick to it, it might be a bit dirty, plus it'll get uneven in spots where it's been worn away by your feet. All these are cues that it's time to clean the old wax off your board and apply new wax.

The easiest way to remove old wax is to leave your surfboard out in the sun for a few minutes (or longer, depending how hot it is) until the wax softens. Then, with the blade edge of your wax comb or an old credit card, start scraping off the wax. Make sure you put newspaper underneath your board when you do this, or do it outside; melted wax can make a mess of the carpet! When you've scraped off all the wax, wipe your board with a cloth to remove any last bits. If there's no sunshine, you can pour hot water over your board, then wipe off the old wax with a cloth. You can also get a wax-removing solvent called Citrus Solve, available at most surf shops. Pour it on and watch the wax come off when you wipe your board clean! When you've got all the old wax off, apply a fresh coat just as you did before, and voilà! A board that looks brand-new!

How to attach your leash to your board

Surf leashes come with a piece of string that threads through a leash plug at the tail of your surfboard. If you thought your leash was the lifeline that connects you to your board, think again. It's actually this tiny piece of string. If it breaks or comes untied, you and your sweet board will part ways. So it's a good idea to be prepared: know how to tie the string, and remember to check that it's secure before you paddle out.

When you have a surf lesson or buy a new surfboard, chances are a leash will already be attached to the board. Many leashes also

SERENA BROOKE: I always check my board after I get out of the water, and sometimes before I go in too, to see if it's got any dings or cracks. If it has, I put [duct] tape over them to stop the rough edges from cutting me, and to stop water from seeping into my board. Stickers also work if you don't have any tape.

✳ tip

If your hands are slimy from sunscreen, grab a handful of wet sand when you get to the water's edge and rub it between your palms until you think you can hold onto your board without its slipping.

have a loop of string sewn into a Velcro strap that attaches to the back of your board so you don't have to tie a knot (until the string breaks). But there will be times when you need to fasten a leash to your board, and that's when it helps to know a few ways to attach the string.

If you've got a leash with a ready-made loop, all you have to do is put one end of the loop under the bar of the leash plug and secure it to the Velcro strap at the skinny end of your leash. (This end is called a "rail saver" because it stops your leash from cutting into the edges, or rails, of your surfboard.) These leashes are great because you don't have to worry about losing that crucial bit of string when you take the leash off your board.

If you're starting from scratch, the easiest way to attach your leash to your board is to make a loop with the string and tie it off with a reef knot or square knot: right over left, left over right. Pull it tight to make sure it's secure; you don't want it to come undone during your next wipeout. Then pass one end of the loop under the bar of the leash plug, bring the two loops together, thread the skinny end of your leash through the double loop, and Velcro it closed.

Don't strap your leash around your ankle until you get to the water's edge—and even then you might want to do some stretches or sit on the sand for a few minutes checking the conditions before entering the water. Putting on your leash is the last thing you do before entering the water.

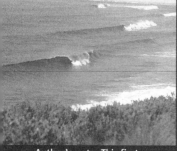

Author's note: This first appeared as an Ask Jodie answer on surfline.com.

JODIE NELSON, PRO SURFER: The secret to finding a good sunscreen for your face (you can use almost anything for your body that's waterproof and has a good SPF rating) is finding one that will stay on in the water and won't clog your pores or sting your eyes. Here's what I do: I start out with a Neutrogena-base liquid sunscreen on my entire face and ears; it's an ultra-sheer dry-touch sunblock with SPF 45. It won't clog pores, it's paba-free, and it's waterproof. It costs about $12 to $16 at most drugstores and grocery stores. Next I apply a brown Shiseido sunblock stick (SPF 35) to my nose, cheeks, and up by my eyes to prevent sunspots and wrinkles. It looks like zinc, makeup or foundation, and it's available at department stores for about $25. Just about every professional surfer I know, male and female, uses Shiseido. Lately, I've been putting it on my forehead as well, because I've noticed a few freckles caused by sun damage. You may think it looks a little silly, but trust me—you'll be happy when you're forty and you don't look like you're sixty!

Getting yourself ready

Face. If you think ahead, you probably applied sunscreen to your face before you left home (to allow it to sink in and to keep it from running into your eyes when you hit the water fifteen minutes from now). If not, now's the time to do it—after you've prepared your board—because touching your board with greasy hands is pretty much a no-no.

Make sure you cover your entire face, including the back of your neck (if you have short hair) and the tops of your ears. I also put sunscreen on the backs of my hands to keep them from getting leathery. I usually put sunscreen on first, wait until it goes in, and then put zinc on my nose and cheeks. Wear a sunscreen with an SPF (sun protection factor) of at least 30. And make sure it's water resistant for at least two hours. Lipstick works really well on lips— it seems to stay on better than a lot of lip balms.

Arms and legs. Remember to put sunscreen on your arms, back, and shoulders if you're not wearing a rash guard. Don't put sunscreen on your legs (except maybe behind your knees—a tender spot) or on your tummy (if you're surfing without a rash guard or wetsuit); standing up is hard enough without a slippery board. There's not much you can do about sun protection for your lower half except to wear long boardshorts.

Hair. If you have long hair, tie it back—if you come to the surface after a wipeout with hair all over your face, it can be hard to get that crucial first breath. Use two elastics if you've got thick hair. Or keep a spare one on your wrist, just in case the one in your hair gets lost out in the water.

Lock it up

One final word before you head off into the blue, leaving your car and all your worldly belongings behind: security. Be careful where you hide your gear or car keys. You'd be surprised how often people watch surfers hide their keys, wait until you're in the water, then, knowing you'll probably be out of sight for at least an hour or two, find the key and drive away in *your* car.

If you're surfing a city beach, don't leave anything on the sand. Lock everything in your car and take your car keys with you out into the water. Most leashes have a pocket inside the Velcro ankle strap, some wetsuits and boardshorts do too (boardshorts often have a string so you can tie your key to them before tucking it into a pocket). Or put the key on a cord around your neck—just make sure you tuck it inside your rash guard or wetsuit so you don't

*tip

If you take your car key out in the water with you, put it in your mouth before you unlock your car to rinse off the salt water and keep the locks rust-free!

WINTER WARMERS

When you surf through winter, or just someplace where the water's always cold, there are a few ways you can make yourself more cozy after your surf.

• If it's a sunny day, hang your towel over your car door while you surf, with its top edge jammed in the closed window. It'll be nicely sun-warmed when you get out of the water.

• When I surfed in Japan, where there are no showers at the beach, I learned a winter survival trick from the local surfers: Fill a large plastic container with hot water before you leave home; by the time you come in from your surf, the water will have cooled enough to be perfect for your own hot shower by the beach!

• Keep a Thermos of hot chocolate in your car for an after-surf treat.

• Give your frozen toes a treat—slip them into a pair of fleecy sheepskin Ugg boots. Mmm . . .

accidentally rip it off and send your key to the bottom of the ocean when you go for your first wave.

Having said all that, some surf spots can be pretty safe. One of my friends, who lives at Montauk, Long Island, regularly leaves her car keys in the ignition while she surfs! So just use your discretion when assessing the safety of a surf spot.

To the beach!

You might have seen surfers running headlong into the surf and jumping right in, and while that can be a good way to warm up your muscles, it's not a good idea for first-timers. For one thing, your board's probably going to be way too big to run with. Taking your time by walking casually to the water's edge also gives you a few minutes to check conditions before you paddle out.

When you're carrying your board down to the water's edge, make sure the wax side is facing out to avoid getting wax on your wetsuit or boardshorts (and taking it off your board, where you need it). This means the fins will be pointing in, so if you have to walk close to anything or anyone, you won't poke them and risk damaging your fins at the same time. (Though some beginners do it, dragging your board along the beach is *not* a good look, and you'll get sand in your wax and damage your board if it hits rocks or other debris hidden in the sand.)

*tip

When carrying your board under your arm, loop your leash over one of the fingers of the hand that's holding your board. Nothing bursts your "Look, everyone, I'm a surfer!" bubble than the old "Oops! I just tripped over my own leash" maneuver.

Stre . . . tch

Unless you'd rather stretch in the privacy of your own home (not to mention on the comfort of your own carpet or yoga mat), it's a good idea to take a few minutes to do some stretches on the sand before you paddle out. It doesn't have to be a big deal—just do what you feel you need.

Stretching warms up your muscles ready for the paddle out, helps to prevent injury, and frees you up so you can surf better. It can be particularly helpful in the early morning when you might be feeling a bit creaky from just rolling out of bed. Stretching on the beach also gives you time to check the waves and decide where to go out. It's quite possible for the conditions to have changed since you first pulled into the parking lot.

How to stretch

You're bound to develop your own routine based on what parts of your body you need to stretch, but for starters here are a few basic moves. Hold each stretch for at least fifteen seconds, breathe in and out deeply (and with each outbreath try to relax into the stretch a little more, feel where it's tight, and try to let the tension go), and make sure you stretch each side equally.

Arms and shoulders. Extend your right arm straight out in front of you, parallel to the ground. Cross your left arm underneath it and hook it with the left elbow. Then pull your straight arm to the left. Good for shoulders. Repeat on other side. Reach one arm up above your head and bend it at the elbow to reach down your back between your shoulder blades. Bring the other arm up to meet it from below, grab on, and feel the stretch in your shoulder joints. Stretch your pecs (the muscles in front of your chest) by clasping your hands together behind your back and lifting up your arms as high as they'll go.

Lower back. Bend forward at the waist to touch your toes, let your arms go floppy, and hang your head like a rag doll. If you can, wrap your arms around the lower half of your legs and pull

YOGA FOR SURFERS

Yoga and surfing go hand in hand. Surfer and yoga instructor Peggy Hall has created a series of fantastic DVDs and videos featuring surf-specific yoga moves that promise to "stretch and strengthen the shoulders, lower back, knees, and hips" as well as prevent injury, improve balance, sharpen your mental focus, and improve your lung capacity and endurance . . . so you can surf better and longer.

What more could a surfer girl want? How about pro surfer Rochelle Ballard demonstrating the moves in front of the surf at Sunset Beach, Hawaii? (See Appendix 3 for contact details.)

YOGA FOR SURFERS with Peggy Hall — featuring Rochelle Ballard & Taylor Knox *Special Edition*

 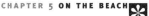

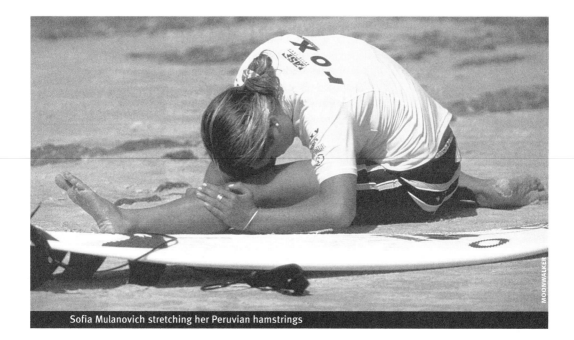

Sofia Mulanovich stretching her Peruvian hamstrings

a little—this will stretch your hamstrings (the backs of your upper legs) as well. Lean forward to put weight on your toes, and lift the muscles above your knees to maximize the stretch. You can also do this stretch sitting down with your legs straight out in front of you. Grab your toes, keep your back straight, and pull gently.

Spinal twists. These are great for loosening up before all that paddling and before the twisting you need to do to turn your board. There are lots of ways to do spinal twists. You can lie on the ground, bend one leg up to your chest, and take it across the opposite side of your body. Or sit up with one leg straight out in front of you, bend the other leg over it, and twist to the side of your bent leg. Hold for several breaths and repeat on the other side.

Hamstrings. Sit on the ground with one leg straight out in front of you and your other leg bent, with the knee pointing out to the side. Keeping your back straight and your hands clasped together, lean forward over your straight leg. Pull your bent leg back a little (don't jerk it, just ease it back), feel where the tension is, and with each outward breath try to relax into the stretch.

Legs. Lean up against a wall or your car as if you were trying to push it over. Keep one leg bent and relaxed and the other (the one you're stretching) straight with the heel on the ground. Or just stand with your hands and feet on the sand and your arms and legs straight, bend one leg and straighten the other, then swap.

Neck. These are pretty straightforward: chin to chest, ear to shoulder, nose to armpit, and then rotate your head in a circle and back the other way.

Quads. For those big muscles on the front of your thighs, stand up, bend one leg, and hold on to your foot behind you. You can also do this lying down: lie on your back and fold both legs under you, trying to relax into the stretch so that your whole body is flat on the ground. You can also stretch your hip flexors by sitting cross-legged on the sand and leaning forward, keeping your back straight. Repeat, with legs crossed the other way.

Are you goofy or regular? (Putting on your leash)

You might have noticed that there are two types of surfers out there: those who stand with their left foot forward (called regular footers, because it was once thought that most surfers stand this way), and those who surf with their right foot forward (goofy footers). Hence the question in surfing circles: "Are you goofy or regular?" (Note: There's no shame in being a goofyfoot).

One of the easiest ways to tell if you're going to be surfing with your right or left foot forward is to find a slippery floor somewhere, put on some socks, take a run-up, and slide across it. Which foot did you put forward? Another way is to get someone

✳ tip

When you're getting out of the surf, don't wind your leash around the tail of your board—the fins can make tiny nicks in the leash, making it more likely to snap later on, probably when you least expect it. Instead, loop it over your board or carry it in your hand.

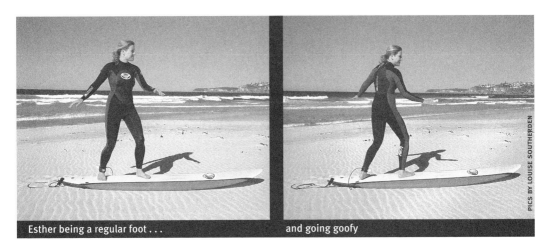

Esther being a regular foot . . .   and going goofy

PICS BY LOUISE SOUTHERDEN

Your ready-for-surfing checklist

Get a beach bag or waterproof surf box (like one of those plastic crates you can buy) that you can keep with your board or leave in the car, containing everything you need for your next surf session. That way you can just grab your surfboard and bag without wasting valuable surfing time getting everything together, or having to stop at the surf shop on the way to the beach because you've forgotten your wax!

Things to put in your surf bag:

- **Surfboard** (just making sure you're paying attention!)
- **Leash** (if it's not already attached to your board)
- Wax and wax comb
- Sunscreen and zinc
- Bikini, boardshorts, rash guard, wetsuit
- Towel
- Sunglasses and hat
- A big bottle of water (to rehydrate and rinse your hair after your surf)
- **Warm clothes** (to put on after surfing)
- **Snacks or loose change** (for the post-surf munchies)
- Optional extras: spare leash and string (in case either one breaks), spare fins (if you have removable fins such as FCS, plus a fin key), spare hair elastics (if you need to keep your hair off your face while you're surfing), leave-in conditioner (to stop your hair from drying out), and tissues (to remove zinc from your nose after your surf).

to stand behind you and give you a shove; whichever foot you put out to steady yourself will be your front foot. And of course, if you ride a snowboard or skateboard you'll already know if you feel more comfortable standing with your left or right foot forward.

Now that you know which way you stand, you also know which ankle to attach your leash to: your back foot. If you're a goofyfoot, your leash goes on your left ankle, and if you're a regular foot, your leash goes on your right ankle.

When you're doing up your ankle strap, make sure the leash extends away from the back of your ankle so you don't trip over it every time you stand up. The strap should be tight enough that it doesn't swivel around, but loose enough to allow you to move your foot freely.

Last words

Remember to relax. Take time to get ready and make sure everything is just the way you like it—sunscreen on, enough wax on your board, leash firmly attached to your ankle. This will help you relax when you're out in the water. And relaxing not only saves you energy and stops you getting tired so quickly, it also allows you to have more fun!

Be aware of your cycles. After a few surfs, you might notice that you surf differently at different times: more gung ho and adventurous some days, more timid and cautious on other days. That's okay. When you understand your own rhythms, you'll be more likely to trust your intuition about when you feel like surfing and when you don't.

Act confident! Confidence comes with practice and with focusing on what you're doing instead of what you look like to others.

PRUE JEFFRIES: I think surfing should be an internal thing in how you approach it. If you concentrate on the little things like where you put your feet or how long your paddling stroke is, it's good for your confidence. Because a lot of the time there's the external factor and that's where girls lose out: they worry about what people think or how they look. The only way you can really overcome that is to focus on what you're doing with your surfing. Don't externalize and worry about what the world thinks and how you look. Just relax.

 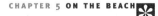

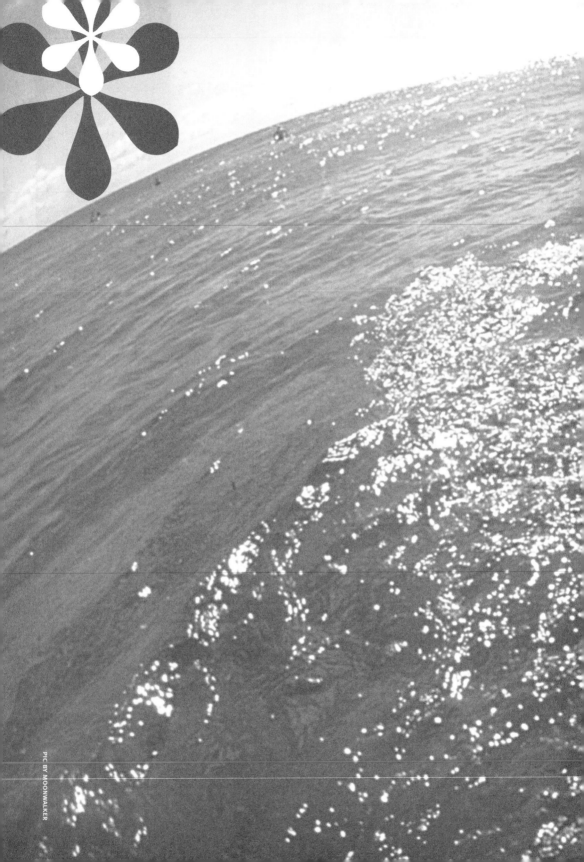

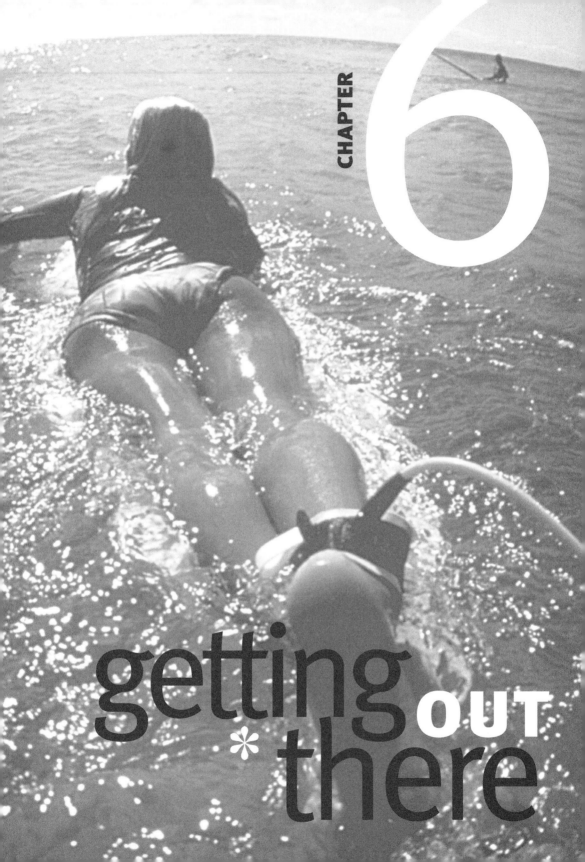

6

getting *out there

Learn:

How to walk your board out into the water. How to paddle out—including lying and sitting on your board, paddling, and tackling the whitewater. **How to do turtle rolls and duck dives.** When to paddle out: the importance of timing. **Where to paddle out: how to use rips.** How to wait for waves and how to turn your board when you're sitting on it.

Welcome to the water's edge! It might not look like much, but you're now standing on hallowed ground: the place where every surfer once stood and wondered, What next? This is where your surfing life really begins. But there's no rush—you've got a lifetime of riding waves ahead of you, and even though you might want that lifetime to start as soon as possible, paddling out is best achieved with a bit of patience.

Walking the walk

Before you can paddle, you have to learn to walk your surfboard out into the water. Even if you think you're beyond this, even if you've lived by the beach all your life, even if you think it just feels silly, walking your board out is a useful skill to learn. Not only does it postpone actually having to paddle your board, it gives you time to get used to the whole concept of being in the water with a foreign object strapped to your ankle. Another advantage of walking your board out is that from a standing position you're higher up—all the better to see the oncoming waves— than if you were lying on your board already.

In fact, even when you become a dedicated surfer, there will be times when you'll still walk your board out. When the water's shallow, it's often easier than paddling. It gives your neck and shoulders a rest. Walking through water also gives your legs a good workout before you start letting your arms dominate. Think of it as your daily aquarobics session!

So, with your leash strapped to your ankle and your board under your arm, walk into the water until it's deep enough to put your board down without letting the fins touch the bottom; waist deep is perfect. Now, with one hand on the deck of your board to keep it from floating away or bumping into you, let your board float *beside you*. Always make sure your board is beside you or on the beach side of you when you're in the water. If it's anywhere else, you're likely to get hit by it when the next set of waves starts marching in.

Stand next to the front of your board so you can lift its nose over each oncoming wave. If the whitewater looks especially big, pick up the board by both rails and lift it cleanly over the wave. When you're ready to catch some whitewater (more on this in Chapter 7), you can also pick up your board and turn it to face the beach before you hop on and ride it in.

Why can't you just push your board out fins first so it's already pointing the right way when you want to catch a wave? Pointing the nose of your board into the oncoming waves lets it ride over

*tip

If you do find yourself between your board and the beach with a wave fast approaching, bob down underwater and leave your board and the wave to battle it out on the surface. Just remember: When you resurface, put your hand up first in case you come up under your board.

them. Besides, when a wave hits a surfboard fins first, the board will turn sideways, and from there it has a pretty good chance of hitting you, the innocent bystander (at this stage).

Paddling out

You might have noticed that the waves you want aren't here where it's shallow, they're *out there* where it's usually too deep to stand—also known as "out the back" (although this technically refers to the place *beyond* the breaking waves). And there's only one way to get there: paddle out.

Paddling out can be one of the most challenging parts of the whole learn-to-surf process. It's exhausting, it seems to take forever, and you're going against what looks like an endless procession of waves whose sole purpose seems to be to wash you back to the beach, where you might think you belong. Don't listen to them! A woman's place is in the waves, not on the sand.

There are three parts to paddling out: lying on your board, paddling your board, and tackling the whitewater.

Lying on your board

Once you're in water that's deep enough—even waist-deep is fine—wait for a break between waves and slide onto your board in a lying-down position. The best place to practice lying on your board is on flat water, so take yourself down to the beach on a day when there aren't any waves or find somewhere calm like a lake, bay, or pool where you can focus on the basics of paddling before you have to think about dealing with bumps in the water—that is, waves.

The secret to balancing on your board is not to lie too far back or too far forward. The nose of your board should be *just* above the surface of the water—a couple of inches at the most. One way to find the balance point on the board is to find where it's not: slide forward, slink back; experiment with different positions on the board and see how they feel. See what happens when you try to paddle. A surfboard moves through the water most efficiently when there's no surfer on it—so slide off your board for a moment and see what it looks like when you're not lying on it. How far is the nose out of the water? This is basically how your board should look when you're lying on it.

Ever seen one of those signs on trains that says KEEP ARMS AND LEGS INSIDE MOVING VEHICLE? It's the same in surfing: When you're lying on your surfboard over the center line (also called the "stringer"), keep those limbs neatly tucked in. Your legs should be

*tip

When you've found out where you should be lying on the board, make a mark of some kind to remind yourself. It can be a sticker that'll line up with your chin or you can make a groove in the wax with your fingernail.

on the board, not splayed out to the side (although that does help your stability at first). The same goes for your arms: even when you're paddling, keep them close to the board.

As you'll soon discover, lying on your board is not nearly as easy or as relaxing as lying on your towel on the beach. For one thing, whenever you're lying on your board, chances are you'll be paddling. You also have to expend some energy keeping your balance on what is essentially an unstable floating object. Keeping your head up and eyes forward to watch for oncoming waves also involves arching your back, lifting your head, and bracing your abdominal muscles to take some of the strain off your lower back.

Paddling your board

Ready to start paddling? I know, it doesn't have quite the glamour of standing up—no one ever says, "Hey, you paddle really well!"— but the truth is that paddling is the backbone of your surfing. You're going to spend more time paddling—paddling out, paddling to catch waves, paddling to stay in position in the lineup— than you are actually riding waves. Not only that, but if you can't paddle strongly you can't catch waves, and if you can't catch waves you can't learn to surf. It's as simple as that.

The best place to learn how to paddle a surfboard is the same place you learned how to lie on it: somewhere with no waves. You can still learn out in the surf, however, in between breaking waves, or when the waves are so small that you can walk your board out past the breakers and paddle around out the back.

How to paddle

Use the same stroke you would use if you were swimming freestyle. Paddle with one arm at a time in long strokes—you don't have to lift your arm very high. Keep your elbow bent and just let it skim above the water. Cup your hands a little and imagine moving water back with each stroke. As one arm is pulling back through the water, the other arm is reaching ahead to get ready.

The biggest mistake beginners make when paddling is to not dig deep enough in the water. Remember, you're not doing this for fun! You're doing it to

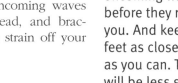

Strong paddling is the key to good surfing

HELP! MY BOOBS GET SQUASHED WHENEVER I PADDLE MY SURFBOARD.

One of the most common mistakes first-time surfers make is to lie with their chests flat on the surfboard when they're paddling, mainly because their back muscles haven't yet developed the strength to hold them off the board. Watch an experienced surfer paddling sometime: She arches her back and lifts her shoulders up off the board so her breasts aren't even touching it (or if they are touching the board, they're not pressing into it). Paddling like this makes your back ache at first, but it also makes paddling much easier: because your shoulders are higher, you won't have to lift your arms so much. It also saves your neck and is more boob-friendly than lying flat.

get past that pesky whitewater, and soon you'll be doing it to catch waves. The more effort you put into each stroke—use your back and shoulders as well as your arms—the fewer strokes you'll need to do. Use this mantra: *long* and *strong*. (That's what your strokes should be like.) Cupping your hands, or separating your fingers a little, can help. Some surfers even use webbed paddling gloves, but you don't really need them, and they can make it harder to hold on to your board.

Once you start paddling, you'll soon find out if you're lying on your board properly. If you're lying too far back, the board will push too much water, making it hard to paddle. If you're too far forward, the nose of your board will start shoveling water with every stroke, which will also slow you down. What you want is for the board to feel like it's cruising along; if you stop paddling, does the board glide for a second or two? If it does, congratulations: You've found your surfboard's sweet spot.

Why paddling a surfboard is so exhausting

The first thing you'll probably notice when you start paddling for any length of time is that it's hard work. There are a couple of good reasons for this. First, even if you're reasonably fit, paddling

ANGIE: I still find the hardest thing is paddling. Not the balance—the first time I lay on a board I didn't fall off or anything. But I guess my upper body strength isn't very good, though it's definitely improved. I just get exhausted. If there's a bit of a current or a rip that's pulling me one way, I end up using all my energy trying to stay in the one spot where I'm trying to catch a wave, and then I don't end up catching any waves because I'm so exhausted from just paddling!

a surfboard uses muscles you didn't know you had—and will probably wish you didn't, by the end of your first day in the water! In particular those muscles at the tops and backs of your arms will suddenly realize with painful clarity that they have a purpose in life.

The second reason paddling feels so hard at first is that you don't yet know the tricks that make paddling out easier:

- You haven't learned how to use rips (riding a rip is the easiest way to paddle out—see later in this chapter).
- You might not be aware of the breaks between sets (experienced surfers often paddle out in these "lulls" instead of struggling against lines of whitewater).
- Your paddling is not as strong as it will be, so it's going to take you longer to get out past the zone of whitewater, and even if you did wait for the lull between sets, chances are it'd be over before you made it out the back anyway. D'oh!

All these lessons come in time, though, and if it's any consolation, you do have one advantage: you're paddling a longboard, which floats more easily and is easier to paddle than a shortboard.

How to get stronger for paddling

The best training for surfing is surfing, but if you can't get out in the water there are other ways to improve your fitness to make paddling a bit easier. Swimming is the most obvious. Saltwater pools are perfect, because the flotation and resistance of seawater feels different from chlorinated freshwater. Laps will help your endurance, but 50-yard or 100-yard sprints will build the power you need for quick bursts of paddling through the whitewater. Imagining that a shark is chasing you is a great way to pick up the pace! Paddling is the aerobic part of surfing—the part where you need good cardiovascular fitness—so anything you can do to improve your fitness will help. When you can't surf, go for a paddle on your board, get out on your bike, take your dog for a walk, go sea kayaking, or do some soft-sand running . . . let the beach be your gym.

Tackling the whitewater

Ah, yes, the old washing machine, the whitewater, the whitewash, the foam . . . whatever you call it, that bubbling fury of "water meets air" can be a formidable obstacle. Even when you're just standing unsuspectingly beside your faithful board in tiny waves,

*tip

The hardest paddle-out is the one before you catch any waves. You haven't loosened up yet, your head's probably still in the parking lot, but most important, you haven't been energized by the waves. Yes, it's true: Catching waves actually gives you energy!

BETHANY: I realize I need to build a bit of upper body strength, so I decided to start doing weights and lots of swimming and more surfing. That helped but when I was surfing today, my friend Jane said, "You're building all the muscles you need right now." And I thought, Cool, I guess I'll just keep doing this!

*tip

When you're waxing your board, put some wax on the sides of your board where you hold it when you turtle roll or duck-dive—it'll give you a better grip and you're less likely to lose your board, or get hit in the face, in the turbulence of the whitewater.

whitewater can sometimes pack enough of a punch to knock you off your feet like a ninepin in a bowling alley. The trick is to be aware so that you know what's coming and develop a couple of techniques to deal with it, because in these early stages you're going to be spending a large part of your water time hanging out in the whitewater.

There's whitewater and there's *whitewater*. The difference lies in the force of the wave; you'll need to use different techniques with different kinds of whitewater. The basic rule of thumb is that the closer you are to where the wave has broken, the more powerful the whitewater is. Here are a few ways to get you and your surfboard safely through the foam:

Push-ups. When the whitewater reaches you, stay lying on your board, make sure it's pointed directly into the oncoming wave, and do a push-up so the whitewater flows between your body and your board. When the wave has passed, lie down on your board again and keep paddling. Good for tackling small weak waves, on any board.

The "keep paddling and hold on" method. Just before the whitewater gets to you, put in a couple of strong paddling strokes for extra momentum and then grab hold of the rails of your board and hang on until the wave passes. Easy! Also good for small waves, on any board.

Turtle rolls. This involves flipping your board upside down (while still holding on to it!) and letting the wave roll over you.

Duck dives. Used on shortboards, that is, surfboards that you can submerge when you put all your weight on them, although some surfers can do a variation of a duck dive with their longboards.

These last two techniques, turtle rolls and duck dives, involve going *under* instead of *over* the oncoming waves. And because they can be used in all conditions, they're the most important, so let's look a bit more closely at how to perform them.

How to do turtle rolls

Because longboards have so much flotation—that is, after all, why you're learning to surf on one—they're almost impossible to push under oncoming waves. Instead, you need to let the whitewater flow over *the bottom* of your board—because the bottom of your board is convex—by flipping your board just before the whitewater gets to you, as follows:

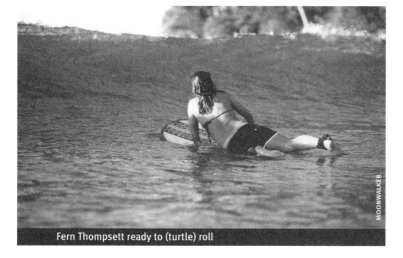

Fern Thompsett ready to (turtle) roll

1. Just before the whitewater reaches you, grab the rails of your board, level with your chest.
2. Holding your board firmly so it doesn't hit you in the face or get wrenched out of your hands by the force of the whitewater, flip yourself and your board upside down so you're underwater (still holding on to your upturned board, hopefully). Oh, yeah: hold your breath for steps 2 and 3.
3. As soon as you feel the wave has passed over you, roll back again to a lying-on-your-board position.
4. Ta-da! You're now ready to start paddling again.

It always amazes me how smoothly even big waves will roll over your board when it's upside down like this. If you hang on, there's not much that can go wrong with this maneuver.

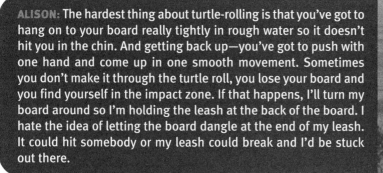

ALISON: The hardest thing about turtle-rolling is that you've got to hang on to your board really tightly in rough water so it doesn't hit you in the chin. And getting back up—you've got to push with one hand and come up in one smooth movement. Sometimes you don't make it through the turtle roll, you lose your board and you find yourself in the impact zone. If that happens, I'll turn my board around so I'm holding the leash at the back of the board. I hate the idea of letting the board dangle at the end of my leash. It could hit somebody or my leash could break and I'd be stuck out there.

 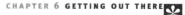

How to duck-dive

Ever seen a duck (okay, a seagull) floating in the surf? When a wave comes, all it has to do is lower its head and let the wave roll right on over its back. That's why we call this move a duck dive. The idea is that you and your board go under the whitewater together and come up when the wave has passed.

You probably won't be duck-diving until you start riding a shortboard—longboards are too hard to push underwater—but if you are learning on a shortboard, or you're thinking of switching to one, it's a useful skill to know.

A perfectly executed duck dive starts before the whitewater hits, goes under all the turbulence (not through it), and brings the surfer (and her board) up to the surface in flat water—ready for the next wave! Here's how to do it, in four easy steps:

1. Paddle right up to the leading edge of the whitewater to give yourself some forward momentum.

2. Just before the whitewater reaches you, grab the rails of your board level with your chest and straighten your arms as if you're doing a bent-knees push-up—except what happens when you start pushing up is that you effectively push your board *down,* under the whitewater. The more buoyant your board, the more you have to push. If you don't push down hard enough, your board won't go under the wave, and you'll get hit in the face with the whitewater.

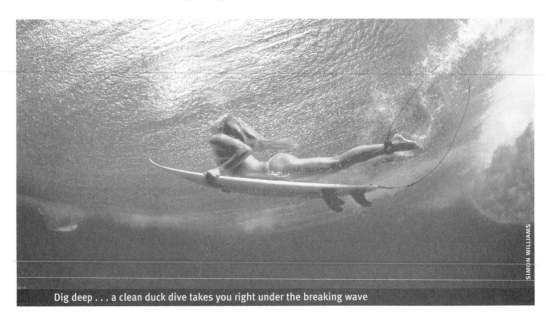

SIMON WILLIAMS

Dig deep . . . a clean duck dive takes you right under the breaking wave

3. Take a deep breath as you and your board submerge, tuck your head down so the whitewater begins to flow over your back, and, as you keep one knee on the back of the board, lift the other leg straight up in the air (preferably the one *not* attached to your leash, although it doesn't matter too much). This gives you the leverage you need to get the nose of your board under the wave.

4. Now the crucial step: surfacing. As with anything sporty, it's all in the knees, or, rather, the knee. As you go under the wave, bring your uplifted leg down and press your other knee into the back of your board to push the tail down. If you don't do this, and you stay in the nose-down-tail-up position, you're making it easy for the wave to push you back toward the beach, just where you *don't* want to be. As the tail of your board goes down, the nose will start to lift up and, if you arch your back a little (think Cobra pose in yoga), you can steer your board back to the surface.

What can go wrong? If you don't push down deep enough, or you pop up too soon, you'll get pummeled by the whitewater. If you don't hold on to your rails firmly enough, or if the wave is just too powerful for your grip, the board can get wrenched out of your hands and hit you or someone else paddling behind you.

Duck-diving sounds more complex than it really is; when you get used to it, it becomes one fluid movement that you do without thinking. With lightweight shortboards it's actually just like diving under a wave when you're bodysurfing. You can even practice pushing your board underwater and bringing it back up, on flat water. The secret is getting your board as deep under the wave as you can: the deeper you go, the farther you are from the churning whitewater.

* tip

If you're not sure you can hold on to your board, try wrapping your legs around it when you're halfway through your duck dive. You'll probably get worked by the whitewater (because you can't go as deep as you can when you duck-dive properly), but at least you won't lose your board and you'll come to the surface sooner than if you'd let it go.

EYES OPEN OR CLOSED?

Duck-diving with your eyes open can be a magical experience when the water's clear and blue. Not only does it look beautiful, it can help you to understand what your board actually does as it goes under the foam: how it tilts down and then tilts back up to the surface. It can also help you to see where the whitewater ends so you know when to bring your board to the surface. There are times, though, when it's not a good idea to open your eyes underwater: if you're wearing contact lenses, of course, or if it's shallow and there's a lot of sand getting stirred up by the waves.

EMY: I get really bloodshot eyes from the surf so I open my eyes underwater only on special occasions like when it's a really glassy wave. I have these moisturizing eyedrops that I keep in my surf bag and I use them before I go in, then after I come out I put more drops in.

Bailing out—the last resort

There is one more technique that surfers use in the whitewater: bailing out or tossing away your board. It's pretty simple: as soon as you realize that you can't turtle roll or duck-dive under the fast-approaching wall of whitewater, you ditch your board, leaving it (and any surfers within range) to face the consequences while you swim under the breaking wave.

When you're learning, it's tempting to throw away your board at the first sign of whitewater—after all, swimming under a wave is a whole lot easier than having to hold on to a big surfboard, stop it from hitting you, and get through the whitewash without drowning. Here are three good reasons *not* to bail:

1. You come up to the surface faster when you're holding on to your surfboard—which is, let's face it, a massive flotation device—than when you're not.

2. Bailing your board is dangerous for surfers and swimmers in your immediate vicinity. If you're riding an 8-foot board and it's got an 8-foot leash, that means you've got a danger zone of more than 16 feet in all directions in which to inflict harm on someone else. If you do discover that you need to bail out, *look behind you first* to make sure there's no one paddling out or swimming nearby. If there is another surfer close enough to get hit by your errant board, try to hang on to your board as best you can; even wrap your legs around it if you have to. Other surfers will respect you for your consideration.

3. In the world of surfing, you're not going to earn much respect if you toss your board at the merest hint of whitewater. Sure, there will be times when you absolutely *must* bail out (see below), but keep it in the BREAK GLASS IN CASE OF EMERGENCY category; it's not an everyday item.

So when is it okay to bail out? There are times, particularly when you're learning, when there will be no other option except to toss your board and dive under the oncoming wave: When the wave in front of you looks too enormous to turtle roll or duck-dive under, when you're scared and don't know what else to do, or when you're just too exhausted to try anything else. Beginners are generally forgiven for bailing, and for this reason other surfers will often give you a wide berth. Return the favor: try to stay out of the way of other surfers. One day you'll be grateful to the beginners who do the same for you.

When to paddle out— the importance of timing

In surfing, as in life, timing is everything. Long before you start catching waves, you'll realize that deciding *when* to paddle out is as important as *where*.

Rule No. 1: Wait for the lull

When the waves are small, you can often just paddle out as soon as you reach the water's edge. But when the whitewater has a bit of a punch to it, it's a good idea to time your paddle-out to coincide with the pause between sets, the lull. This is a good time to paddle out because you won't have to tackle so much incoming whitewater.

When you're standing at the water's edge, watch the waves coming in and look for the pauses. When it looks like there's going to be a break in the waves, start walking out into the water. By the time the last wave of the set has broken and made its way to where you're standing, you'll be ready to go.

Rule No. 2: Find your moment and go!

The best way to use timing to your advantage is to paddle out quickly—although that's easier said than done. Just try to focus on a spot you want to reach and keep paddling to make the most of the lull between waves.

WHITEWATER-FREE ZONES
Paddling out is not always white and foamy. Sometimes, because you timed it right or you just got lucky, you get to paddle out over unbroken waves—all you have to do is keep paddling—or through breaking waves. If the oncoming wave is just about to break, you can push the nose of your board through the face of the wave.

LOATA: I used to just go for it, I'd never wait for the waves to die down, then I'd be stuck in the whitewash trying to duck-dive this very buoyant board. It'd take me half an hour just to get out. I remember Colin, my husband, saying to me, "Wait until it calms down and then you'll just power through." And rips are so helpful. It's amazing how easy paddling out can be when you know where to go. I haven't had the guts to jump off the rocks yet, but that's my dream.

Where to paddle out

Some days the waves will keep marching in one after the other, and on those days *where* you paddle out will be more critical than *when*. So where should you paddle out?

Most of the time when you're surfing at a beach break, you won't have a lot of choice; it's just a matter of picking a spot where the waves aren't dumping too much, maybe somewhere they're a little smaller and the whitewater doesn't look like a set of Grade 5 rapids.

There are two main options for paddling out with the least amount of effort:

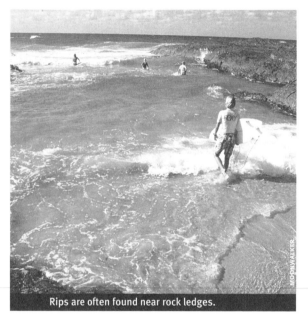

Rips are often found near rock ledges.

First look for a rip, often found near rocks, that will carry you through the whitewater faster than you can say, "How did I get out here so fast?"

And if there are no rips, see if you might be able to jump off the rocks to get to the lineup, instead of paddling through line after line of whitewater.

Using rips to paddle out

Put simply, a rip is a channel where the current is moving out to sea. Wherever you get waves breaking on a beach, there will generally be a rip. On long beaches especially, the water that's surging toward the shore needs to get back out to the ocean, so it digs channels in the sandy bottom and runs out, carrying happy surfers (and hapless swimmers) with it.

ALISON: If you don't know where to paddle out, like if you're at a strange beach and you've been standing there watching the surf for ten minutes and you still don't know, look for people who are catching waves in and see where they paddle back out. The other day we went to a beach where we hadn't surfed before so I walked up to the lifeguard and said, "I've never surfed here before, where do you suggest I paddle out?" And he said, "Over by the rocks, you can't tell from here but there's a rip over there, you can use that."

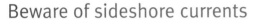

LOATA: When I went to Byron Bay, Australia, the waves were beautiful and the girl I was with was saying "C'mon, let's go, let's go!" but we were new there; we didn't know the beach at all. And I saw this old guy, all leathery and brown, so I asked him, "Is it safe to surf over there where it's breaking beautifully?" And he said, "No, the current is too strong—if you catch a wave you'll be in the danger spot, and it's really tough to get yourself out of there." So it's a good idea to ask the locals.

Beware of sideshore currents

While currents that take you out to the break can help you paddle out, currents that go along the beach—called sideshore, longshore, or littoral currents—can be dangerous. You might not realize you're drifting, but you'll get tired and you can end up miles away from where you started. Watch other surfers paddling out and make a mental note of where you left the beach to see if you're drifting. Also, when you're waiting for waves and you have to keep paddling to stay in position, your surf session is effectively halved because you don't get the usual rest time between riding waves.

Jumping off the rocks instead of paddling out

Once you've mastered the art of getting through whitewater head-on, you'll discover that at some surf spots you can bypass the whitewater altogether by jumping off the rocks into deep water and paddling over to the lineup.

Some surfers routinely jump off the rocks to get to the takeoff spot, particularly at their local break where they probably know every nook and cranny in the rock platform they leap from. Others use it mainly as a big-wave option when it's virtually impossible to paddle out through the whitewater. Either way, it has definite advantages. It gets you out to the lineup sooner, you don't use up as much energy paddling out, and it puts you right into the takeoff spot so you can start catching waves as soon as possible.

Timing is everything when you're launching yourself off the rocks. The aim of the game is to stand on the edge of a rock platform at water level, with your board under your arm and your leash on, waiting for the right moment to leap into the water with your board in front of you so that you're ready to start paddling as soon as you hit the water. Watch the sets for as long as you need to (it can take a while to get the rhythm of the waves). Often, just

*tip

Paddling out is as much a mental challenge as a physical one. Even experienced surfers have days when they can't get through the whitewater—the waves are too big or too relentless, there's too much current—and it can be discouraging. A healthy dose of determination can help, but it's important to know when to turn around and come back to the beach. Sometimes, if you have a rest and watch the waves a bit more, you can see an easier spot to go out.

after the biggest wave of the set, there'll be a brief window—like the lull in the whitewater when you were paddling out from the beach. Then you can jump, letting the surge off the rocks carry you back out with it. Watch where other (experienced!) surfers jump, too, so you can see where the best spot is.

What can go wrong? There are several reasons surfers often prefer a slog through whitewater than a risky leap of faith: goof up and the consequences can be dire. You can trip on your leash as you're running along the rocks (always loop it over the fingers of the hand carrying your board). You can slip on wet rocks or get your foot caught in a rock pool or crevice in the rock platform. You can mis-time the sets and get washed back onto the rocks. Or you can misjudge the depth of the water when you jump and throw yourself onto barely submerged rocks—ouch!

Ready and waiting

Now that you've made it out past the whitewater and into the lineup (so called because it's where waiting surfers often form a line), you've earned a rest. This is one of the most enjoyable parts of surfing: sitting out the back on your surfboard, waiting for waves.

Sitting on your board

*tip

Sitting astride a surfboard is similar to sitting on a horse: there's motion in all directions and you have to use your hips to balance. Try to bring your center of gravity down to your belly—relax your shoulders and try not to hold on to your board with your hands. Just use your feet and your hips to stay upright.

Sit up on your board facing the direction of the oncoming waves. It'll give your back a rest after all that paddling, and it also gives you the advantage of height: You can see farther and therefore see waves sooner, which gives you more time to turn your board around and get ready to start paddling for them.

Here's yet another reason to learn to surf on a big board rather than on a toothpick (as short pointy boards are commonly called): They're easier to balance on. Because they're bulky, longboards are more stable, not just when you're paddling and riding them, but when you're sitting on them as well. Having said that, sitting on any floating object in the ocean takes some getting used to. Use your legs for balance—you can even swirl your feet in circles to keep from falling off (it does wonders for your ankles!). This is also a good way to turn your board around when you see a wave you want to catch.

Getting your bearings

When you get out the back, there won't be any more waves to turtle roll under, so you can relax a bit and have a look around.

Where are you in relation to the beach? In relation to the breaking waves? Where are all the other surfers waiting for waves? Are there any surfers paddling out or sitting near enough to you to get in the way when you decide to paddle for a wave?

Conditions in the water can change suddenly and without warning. One minute you're sitting in the right spot to catch a wave, the next you've drifted into a channel where no waves are breaking.

Next time you're out in the water, take a moment to notice where you are in relation to the shore and line yourself up with a landmark on the beach so you will be able to tell if you start drifting. It can be anything: a house, your car, a tree that sticks up a bit more than the ones around it, even your towel on the sand. At some surf spots, you need to get two reference points on the land: one directly in front of you on the beach and one to the side so you can see if you start drifting out as well as along the beach.

Turning your board around

Although you need to sit facing the open ocean to watch for any waves coming your way, you'll need to be facing the beach when the time comes to catch one. This means you're going to have to turn your board around.

Turning your board 180 degrees while lying on it is not only slow, it's awkward. The only thing you should be doing when you're lying on your board is paddling.

Turning your board around from the sitting position is much easier. Use your hands in the water and swirl those feet. Turn your torso in the direction you want to go. Or lean back on your board so the nose lifts out of the water a bit; then you can pivot around on the tail of your board, which is easier than trying to drag the whole board through the water.

Give yourself plenty of time to turn around at first, but what you're aiming for is speed. The faster you can turn your board around, the sooner you'll be catching waves. In fact, next to paddling, turning your board around quickly is the single most important thing you can do to prepare yourself for catching waves. So practice sitting on your board, even on flat days or in a lake or pool; practice turning to the left, to the right, 180 degrees, and full circle in both directions; and aim to do it quickly and fluidly. Before you even think about catching waves, you need to be able to turn your board at a moment's notice because that's often all the warning you'll get when a wave you want is bearing down on you!

* tip

Wait for waves with your board at an angle to the beach— that way you won't need to turn your board through a complete half-circle. If you know which way the next wave is going to break, even better: if it's a right-hander, you can angle your board to the right so you're ready to start paddling that way; vice versa for a left-hander.

Last words

Don't give up! This is not supposed to be discouraging, but beginner surfers have the toughest time of anyone in the water and that can be physically and mentally exhausting ("Why can't I do this?"). If it's any consolation, the more you surf, the easier it is to paddle out—but no one gets through this process without a bit of struggle. Think of it as a rite of passage, a kind of "baptism of foam."

Make friends with your fear. That's easier said than done when you're attached to an 8-foot hunk of foam that seems more foe than friend and when you're in unfamiliar aquatic territory, but that's all the more reason to calm down and take it easy. Particularly when you're new to surfing, nothing saps your energy faster than feeling scared and fearful. We've all been there. It's a completely normal part of learning to surf.

Never turn your back on the ocean. This probably sounds like something your parents drummed into you as a toddler, but you know what? They were right. The sea can be downright unpredictable. You don't have to be paranoid about it; just pay attention. When you get a feel for the ocean and the waves, you can relax this rule—but by then you'll be fixing your gaze on the horizon for another reason: so you don't miss that next wave!

Help each other. Even when you're a beginner and you think you don't know anything worth passing on, don't undervalue what you've learned so far. You might surprise yourself.

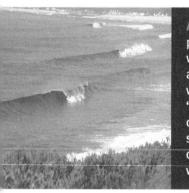

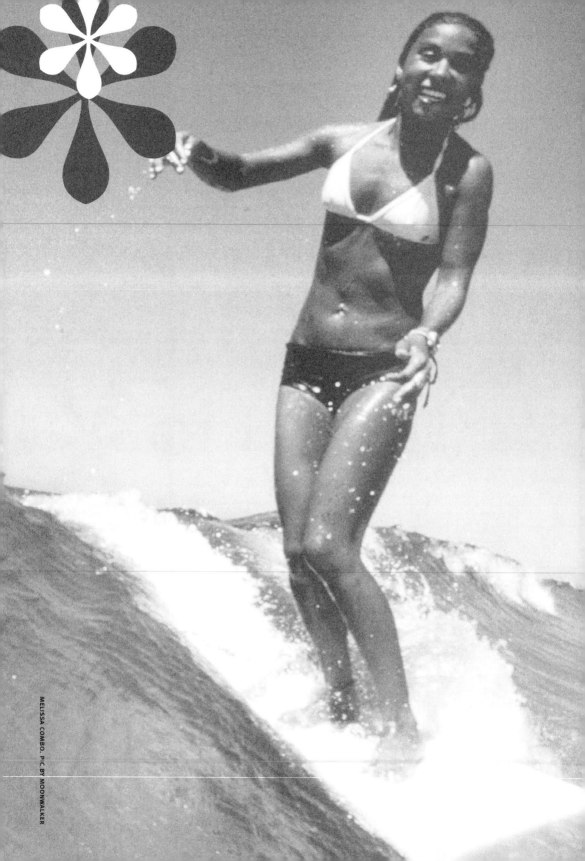

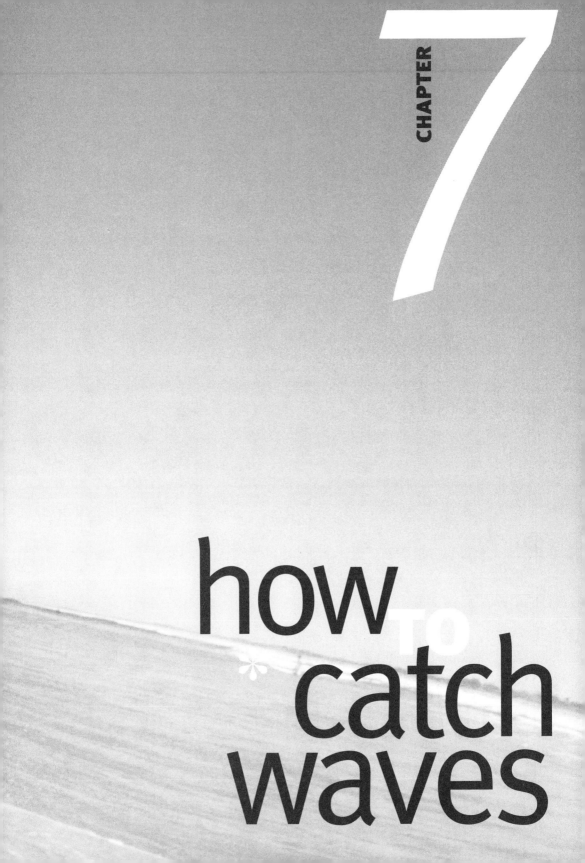

how **to** catch waves

Learn:

How to ride whitewater. **How to paddle for breaking green waves.** How to take off on a wave. **The three keys to standing up on a (moving!) surfboard.** Things that can go wrong—and how to avoid them. **The art of wiping out.**

✳

Watch an experienced surfer take off on a wave sometime. There she is, sitting on her board with her back
to the beach. She sees a wave coming, nonchalantly
turns her board around, and starts paddling for it.
Then, at just the right moment, she springs effortlessly to her feet
and cruises down the face of the wave like she's been doing this
all her life. And she may have been—although it's more likely that
she learned how to catch waves just like you're about to do.

Catching the whitewater

You've learned a multitude of skills to get out past the whitewater,
but now that you're ready to start catching waves, it's a good idea
to start back in the foam.

Why start in the whitewater?

Basically, it buys you some time before you have to think about
all the tricky things like timing, positioning, and how to stand up.
It also helps by:

- Giving you a feel for what it's like to catch a wave. Getting
an intuitive sense of what it feels like when the wave has
picked you up will help hugely when you start catching breaking "green" waves.
- Giving you a feel for how your fast-moving surfboard responds to different movements; it's also a safe place to
experiment.
- Relaxing you. Because you're riding a wave that's already
broken, timing is not an issue so all you have to do at this stage
is point your board for the beach, hop on, and hold tight . . .
and the wave will carry you and your board safely to shore.

Apart from all that, it's fun! Surfing's supposed to be fun, right?
Don't worry, you'll soon get to the frustrating part of catching
green waves, so enjoy the ride while it's still easy!

Launching yourself into waves

Standing in shallow water, hold your board beside you and wait
for a lull between waves. This is your window of opportunity for
getting in position to launch yourself into your first wave. When
you're ready, turn your board around so it's pointing toward the
beach, lie down, and start paddling. You won't have to paddle
much at this stage; if you're in the right position on your board,

✳**tip**

How can you tell if
the wave's got you?
The tail of your board
will lift up, and you'll
feel yourself surge
forward. If you
paddled for the wave,
it's the point at
which you can stop
paddling and start
enjoying the ride.

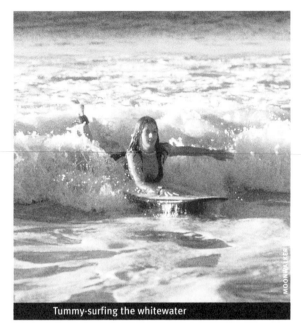

Tummy-surfing the whitewater

the whitewater will just collect you on its way to the beach.

Do this a few times, and try each time to pinpoint the exact moment when the wave has you in its grasp. Saying something to yourself like "Now!" is a good way to remember to watch for it.

Tummy-surfing

Don't worry about standing up yet—there'll be plenty of time for that later. Besides, you've got enough to do right now. While you're lying on your board enjoying the ride, tune in to what's going on. Can you feel the wave losing power as it gets closer to the beach? What happens when you lean left or right? Grab the rails and try moving the board around; zigzag to the beach if you can.

Shuffle back on the board a bit, forward a bit—what's happening now? This is a good time to check your positioning. If you keep nosediving when you've caught the wave, you're probably lying too far forward on the board; if the wave just washes right over you, you're probably too far back.

A few womanly hazards

While we're still in the whitewater, it's probably a good idea to fill you in on a few, shall we say, uncomfortable aspects of being a female surfer:

✳tip

When you ride the whitewater, try to stop before the fins hit the sand—softboards with rubbery fins won't mind too much, but fiberglass boards, with fins that can snap off, will.

● **Red and raw.** They don't call them rash guards for nothing. If you're just wearing a bikini—that is, no rash guard or wetsuit—lying on those softboards you see at all the surf schools can give your bare belly a bit of a rash. Unfortunately, there's not much you can do except wear a rash guard or wetsuit until you graduate to a smoother fiberglass board, or until you develop thicker skin on your belly! You can also get red marks or bruises where the tips of your ribs or the front of your hips press into the surfboard when you're lying on it. A wetsuit top or wetsuit will give you a bit of padding.

● **Nipple rash.** The flatter you lie, the more pressure on your breasts and the more your nipples will rub on the deck of your surfboard, particularly when you're cold. Try arching your back when you're paddling, and stay warm!

● **Jangly jewels.** Jewelry can definitely get in your way—some rings can prevent your getting a good grip on your board when you're duck-diving or doing a turtle roll, bangles can make your hand slip off the board when you go to push up, and necklaces can get caught in your fingers as you stand up. The same goes for the strap at the top of the zipper on your wetsuit: If you find it's getting in your way, tuck it into the neckband of your wetsuit. Toe rings don't seem to cause too much of a problem, but belly-button rings and studs definitely can.

Paddling for broken waves

Once you've mastered launching yourself into waves and tummy-surfing, it's time to start paddling for those same broken waves—that is, the whitewater. Here goes:

1. Sitting on your board, facing out to sea, pick an approaching wave and make a decision to go for it.
2. Turn your board around while you're sitting on it, and, when it's pointing toward the beach, lie down and start paddling.
3. Keep an eye on the wave by looking back over your shoulder. Timing isn't as critical as when you're going for breaking waves (see below), but you still don't want to be too far in front of the whitewater because it'll lose momentum once it's broken and the ride won't be as much fun. Remember, the closer you are to where the wave breaks, the more power it will have.
4. Paddle, paddle, paddle and only stop when you're sure the wave has picked you up.
5. Hang on to your rails and ride the wave in to the beach.
6. You can try standing up now if you want to, but bear in mind that it's bumpier riding the whitewater than riding breaking waves.

Catching breaking (green) waves

Now comes the tricky part: catching waves that haven't broken yet—or, more accurately, catching waves *as they break*. Timing and positioning are everything. The aim of the game is to match the speed of the wave with your paddling, so your board needs some momentum before the wave gets to you. The hardest thing is trying to keep up with the wave. It's rare that anyone will paddle too *fast* when they're starting out—although it can happen and in that case, you'll end up way out in front of the wave and will be riding the whitewash again. More often, you won't be paddling hard enough, and the wave will just sail on by without you.

How to paddle for waves

The thing that distinguishes surfing from almost any other activity you will ever learn is the movement—not only are you moving (or soon will be), but the environment is constantly moving too. That's why there's so much to pay attention to and why when you're learning, it feels as if everything is happening so fast. One minute you're looking at an oncoming wave and deciding whether to catch it, and the next you're floundering in the whitewater wondering what went wrong. It's all part of the learning process, but it might help to break this seamless move into its component parts:

- **Pick a wave, any wave.** Knowing which wave to catch is the first step—have another look at Chapter 4 to remind yourself of the kinds of waves you want. Basically, they should be small and not too steep. Now look around and find the peak—that is, where the waves are breaking—and then find a wave you think you can catch.
- **Turn around and start paddling.** Remember you're going to be sitting on your board when you first see the wave. So turn your board around in this sitting position and, when it's pointing in the direction you want to go, lie down and start paddling. You might have to paddle toward the wave before you start paddling for the beach—just to meet it where it's going to break. Anticipating a wave's movements is something that comes with time, but you can give yourself a head start by watching other surfers.
- **Paddle hard!** The more effort you put into paddling, the less paddling you'll have to do. The hardest strokes will be at the beginning, to get your board going, but once it's moving, if you keep up the pace you'll find yourself moving pretty swiftly.

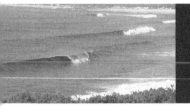

- **Give yourself plenty of time.** The advantage of riding a bigger board is that you can catch waves before they get too steep, but this means you might have to start paddling earlier than other surfers riding shorter boards.
- **Look back over your shoulder** as you paddle, to check on the wave's progress. Then you can slow down or speed up your paddling, or paddle closer to where it's going to break (or farther away from it!), to make sure you'll be in the right position to catch it.
- **Don't stop paddling until you're sure you've caught it.** This is the key to paddling onto breaking waves. If in doubt, do a couple of extra strokes just to be sure.

The PLF method

One of my friends was learning to surf at Manly Beach in Sydney recently, and this older guy, seeing her wipe out yet again on the takeoff, paddled over and proffered this advice: "You need to learn the PLF method," he said coolly. I looked on, wondering what on earth he was talking about. Then he explained: "PLF: paddle like f——!" He was right: When you're paddling for a wave, give it all you've got. The most common mistake beginners make when paddling for waves is they don't paddle hard enough—so the waves overtake them and they end up feeling like a bit of debris bobbing around in the lineup.

Paddle on an angle

When you first start paddling for waves, you'll point your board straight at the beach. Later on, when your paddling gets a bit more sophisticated, you'll be able to predict which way the wave is going to break—right or left (see below)—and paddle for it on an angle. This saves you from having to turn your board completely around in the sitting position, lessens the risk of nosediving, and also makes the takeoff easier if you're at an angle when you stand up. Just beware of angling your board too sharply along the face of the wave; your board might flip and send you flying. Game over.

Right or left?

This is a good question to ask before you catch a wave, because you'll need to know which way you're going to be riding the wave so you can paddle right or left and, any moment now, ride the wave in the direction it's breaking.

∗tip

Lean forward when you're paddling for a wave. The more weight you have forward at this critical stage, the more likely you are to catch the wave. The trick is in knowing when to bring your weight back so your board doesn't nosedive.

Whether to go right or left is partly up to the wave: some waves break right, some break left, and some you can ride either way (they're called A-frame peaks because they look like a capital *A* and break right and left simultaneously, allowing one surfer to ride to the right, and another to the left). And it's partly up to you: whether you feel more comfortable riding a right-hander or a left-hander (more about this in Chapter 9).

Taking the drop, taking off

One thing that unhinges most surfers when they come to catching breaking waves for the first time is the fear of taking the drop: that is, going down the face of the wave. And for good reason. Although this is where all the glory happens ("Nice takeoff" being one of the sweetest compliments a girl can hear) and where you feel the rush of catching a wave, it's also the most vulnerable position on the wave.

This is where the wave's energy is most intense. They don't call it the "impact zone" for nothing. Which means the consequences of making a mistake on your takeoff are greater than at any other time. Your board can nose-dive and send you flying. You can fall off and hit your board; you can fall onto your board. The lip can break on top of you. Falling off at this point, while it happens to the best of us, is likely to have consequences. It might not hurt—after all, you're not in shallow water anymore—but it might be scary for a while.

A word about commitment

Ah, yes, the c-word. While it'd be nice to say that every time you paddle for a wave, you should commit to taking it, it doesn't always work that way. There will be times when you start paddling

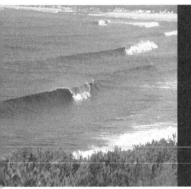

ALISON: The thing about catching unbroken waves is you have to make yourself do it. And one way to do that is if you and your girlfriends take turns pushing each other onto waves . . . it's fantastic. When I was learning to surf, my coach Gally took me out the back and said, "You're going to go for this wave," and he pushed the back of my board and I had no option but to jump up and ride it because I was too frightened of falling off! Just a gentle shove is often enough to get you up there, and once you know the joy of catching those waves, you're much more comfortable paddling back out and doing it yourself.

for a wave and then decide at the last minute not to go for it. It might be too steep, it might be a closeout (not breaking left or right, but collapsing along its length, leaving no space to ride it), or you might realize that you're not ready to throw yourself to the lions just yet.

This is called "backing off" (or "chickening out," in some circles), and it has consequences:

● Other surfers might start encroaching on your waves (dropping in on you) if they think you're not going to catch the waves you paddle for.
● It can scare you more to back off a wave than to go for it—our minds are so clever, they can invent all kinds of scenarios in the space of a millisecond. Wiping out is rarely as bad as you imagine.
● If you back off the wave too late, you can get sucked over anyway in the time-honored beginner's maneuver, "going over the falls," so-called because it's like going over a waterfall head first with your board. And if you think that's bad, consider this other variation: going over the falls while *sitting* on your board. Although you're paddling for the wave, at the point where you back off, you'll probably sit up and lean back on your board—but, alas, not soon enough. It won't be one of your proudest moments, but your friends will probably thank you for the amusement!

Standing up

Now, the moment you've been waiting for, the moment when you can, at last, stand on a surfboard and call yourself a real surfer!

Three things to remember:

1. **One movement.** The key to your "pop-up" or "jump-up" is standing up in one smooth movement, so that you can do it quickly. The less time you spend in transition from lying to standing, the less time there is to mess up the takeoff and the sooner you can start riding the wave.

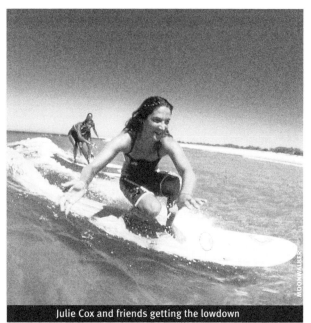

Julie Cox and friends getting the lowdown

142

✳ How to practice pop-ups on the beach

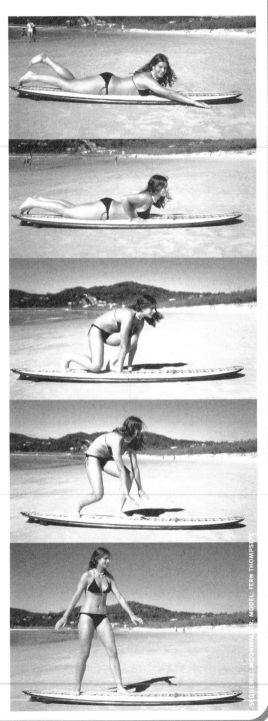

1. Paddle for the wave, looking over your shoulder at the wave behind you.

2. Put your hands flat on the board and start to push up.

3. As you push yourself up, bring your feet underneath you.

4. Stand up but stay low. Keep your hands low for balance.

5. If you're feeling confident, straighten up a little. Note foot placement: front foot angled, back foot across the board.

SEQUENCE: MOONWALK. MODEL: FERN THOMPSETT

Izzy Tihanyi, Surf Diva: You don't have to pop up like a "jack in the box." It's better to do controlled, smooth pop-ups: head and shoulders up first, look where you're going, and don't forget to smile!

2. **No knees.** It's tempting to take a shortcut through kneesville on your way to your feet. This might be how you'd get up from lying on the floor at home, but it's not how you get up on a surfboard. Don't do it. Getting to your knees makes the board more unstable and will slow down your pop-up.

3. **Stay low.** Don't be in a hurry to straighten up once you're on your feet; it's the quickest way to ensure you don't stay up very long. Bend your knees, tuck your bottom in, and keep your hands down (you can even hold on to your board until you get your balance), or put them out to the side like airplane wings. Cool!

On the beach

The best way to get an idea of what you're going to be doing out in the water is to do it on land first (see full-page box). So practice standing up on your board while you're on the beach. Put your board down. Make sure the fins are stuck in the sand and not over any rocks or other hard objects, or take out the fins (if they're removable) for this step. Now, lie down on your board, look over your shoulder, and start paddling for a pretend wave.

Jump up!

Standing up on a surfboard is as easy as one, two, three—at least in theory. In practice, it's all about practice!

1. Put your hands flat on the deck of the board, level with your chest, and push your body up over your hands, keeping your feet on the board.

2. Now swing your legs up under you so you're kinda crouching over the centerline (marked by the stringer) of your board. The knee of your front leg will be under your chest. Your back foot will probably tilt onto its side—that's okay, it'll straighten when you stand up.

3. Let go of your board with your hands and stand up, using your legs to balance. Make sure your weight is over the centerline (the stringer) of your board, evenly distributed between both feet. Leaning too far forward isn't usually a problem—in fact, that can help you to balance at first. But if you lean too far back (a common boo-boo), you'll fall off the back of the board.

There you have it! Standing upright, knees bent with your feet a bit wider than hip width apart and your arms out to the side or down low for balance. Your back foot will be across the board and your front foot will be angled slightly toward the nose.

*tip

Practice doing at least ten pop-ups on the floor every night—it'll train your body to do it smoothly.

What can go wrong?

Standing up too early. You paddle for the wave, think you've caught it, and just when you get to your feet . . . you find the wave has passed underneath you, and you're left standing on your board, sinking feet first into flat water. The trouble is that when you stand up, a lot of your weight goes to the back of your board—but putting weight at the front of the board helps you to catch the wave.

Solution: Make sure you've caught the wave before trying to stand up. Take a few more strokes when you're paddling for it and lean forward so you almost push your board down the face of the wave. Only stand up when you're sure you've caught the wave.

Standing up too late. You're at the bottom of the wave, you've lost all speed, and, as one of my friends says, "It's like trying to ride a bicycle very, very slowly" (more unstable and difficult than it needs to be). Plus, you're in rather a precarious position: The wave is about to break on top of you.

Solution: You need to get to your feet more quickly. Practice pop-ups at home and try to get up as quickly as you can. And when you're catching waves, try to do your pop-up as soon as you know you've caught the wave.

Pearling. An elegant word for what is basically a very awkward experience: nose-diving; this is when the nose of your board careers down the face of the wave so steeply that it keeps on going, burying itself in the water and sending you anklet over belly button into the air. It might happen because the wave is simply too steep for your longboard, or because you're standing or lying too far forward on your board.

Solution: When you're on a wave and you feel the nose of your board heading down and threatening to start shoveling water, lean back and put all your weight at the back of your board. This way,

✳ **tip**

Standing up will be so much easier if you have strong legs. Practice doing knee bends at home, or the Warrior yoga pose. Running, bike riding, and swimming with a kickboard will also help.

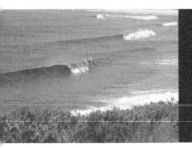

ALISON: When I started surfing, I had a lot of trouble jumping up. Then one day I was wearing red nail polish on my toes, and when I came out of the surf there were red streaks up and down my board and I thought, Bingo! So now I pretty much always wear red toenail polish and if I come back from a day's surfing and there's millions of streaks, I know I've been dragging my toes and I haven't done clean jump-ups.

taking the drop is like riding an elevator; you're going down but you're standing on a horizontal surface that, if you can control it, will take you down safely. If it's a wave-selection problem, try to pick waves that aren't so darn steep. It can be difficult to see how the waves break when you're sitting out the back, so make the most of the view when you're paddling out; you'll have a perfect vantage point to see the face of the waves. Take a look along the beach, too; there might be a spot where the waves aren't breaking so steeply and you can try surfing over there.

Taking too long to get to your feet. If you take too long to get to your feet, chances are the wave will start breaking and you'll be stuck behind the whitewater. Waves don't wait for anybody, so you'll need to practice getting to your feet as fast as you can—on land if necessary.

Solution: It might be hard to believe, but Layne Beachley had this very problem even when she started competing on the pro tour. Here's how she handled it: "I'd developed this weird two-step routine where I'd get one foot on the board and then the other, which was pretty annoying. I was ranked number two in the world and I couldn't even stand up properly! But bad habits can always be remedied. I used to take the fins out of my board, lie it on my bed, and practice springing up on both feet at the same time. I also practiced jump-ups on the floor of my room, over and over again. It worked!"

Wipeout!

At this stage of your surfing life, you're likely to be spending a fair amount of time in what we like to call "the dismount." Someone once told me that if you're not wiping out, you're not really trying. There's some truth in that—if you're afraid to fall off, you'll be afraid to try new moves.

Wiping out may be an art form, but because it involves being underwater where, last time I checked, you can't breathe, it's important to know how to do it safely:

● Try to fall away from your board, preferably into the white-water, the safest part of the wave.

● Remember the talk about bailing your board? The same applies when you wipe out: your board becomes a missile with a range of about 16 feet (that's 8 feet of board plus an 8-foot leash), so beware of other surfers paddling out or in your way when you wipe out and do everything you can to stop your board from

tip
Focus on your back foot. When I was learning how to stand up, one of my friends told me not to worry about where I was putting both feet when I stood up—instead, he said, focus on getting your back foot in place. If you put weight over the back foot when you're taking off, it also stops you from nose-diving.

EMY: If I'm close to the bottom when I wipe out, I always try and push off to get back to the surface. And don't try to come up so you look like a beautiful mermaid with your hair back—you've got to cover your face in case someone's board is coming toward you and they haven't seen you.

✳tip

When you're underwater waiting to come up, see if you can feel your board pulling on your leash. This will give you a clue about where your board is in relation to you and which direction to be wary of when you surface.

ALISON: A lot of surfing comes down to not thinking too much. Gally, my coach, once said to me: "Be where you are." Don't think about the next wave, don't think about the last wave, don't think about your boyfriend or your shoes or what you're having for dinner tonight. Surfing is all about being in the moment.

hitting them or their board (at least until third-party surfboard insurance is invented). If you can, hang on to your board as you fall, so it's at least close to you instead of flailing about in the impact zone, but not if it's going to endanger you.

● When you resurface after being underwater, come up with one hand above your head (both hands wrapped around your head is even better), to protect yourself if your board hits you. Leashes are stretchy, so the impact of losing your board doesn't dislocate your ankle/knee/hip (check one), but the side effect is that your board can "slingshot" back at you if the leash is overstretched.

● If you're in shallow water, fall shallowly. That is, don't dive head-first; flop into the water instead, and spread your arms and legs out like a starfish to stop yourself from hitting the bottom.

● One of the worst parts of wiping out is being held under by the wave. Learning to hold your breath will help, as will training yourself to relax underwater. Most important, don't panic or you'll use up more air and need to come up sooner. Kick off the bottom if you need to, open your eyes underwater so you can see how far away the surface is, and wait for the wave to release you.

Last words

Just do it. One of the great things about surfing, particularly for those of us who spend a good deal of our lives thinking, is that it gets you out of your head for a while. Sure you need to think about weather conditions and where to surf and what you want to practice the next time you paddle out, but once you're out in the water, the best thing you can do is let go. Surfing is, after all, play. Let your natural instincts guide you.

Slow down. In the beginning you'll probably feel as if everything's happening at the speed of light—so fast you can't pay attention to it all: the wave, your surfboard and where it is on the wave, your body, timing, the wind and tides. Don't worry about it. Just focus on each step as it happens.

Watch videos. Now that you've discovered the great oceanic outdoors, it's time to head back indoors: find as many surfing videos as you can and watch them over and over. Simply watching other surfers rewires your brain so it will know what to do next time you're out there. Or find a friend with a video camera and ask her to shoot you surfing: You'll progress ten times faster because you'll be able to see what you're doing and can correct any bad habits the next time you go out.

Go at your own pace. Learn to surf with your friends, but don't fall into the trap of comparing your progress to theirs. Just because someone else is standing up before you are doesn't mean you won't be a competent surfer. On the flip side, if you're getting the hang of it faster than your friends, keep it in perspective. Sure, standing on a surfboard is the greatest feeling known to woman-kind, but don't let it go to your head. Maybe you can even help your friends or take turns watching each other and giving each other feedback.

Enjoy the journey. We've all heard this before: It's not the destination it's the journey—the journey across the wave, the journey from beginner to competent surfer. The great thing about surfing is that the journey is fun!

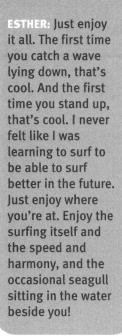

ESTHER: Just enjoy it all. The first time you catch a wave lying down, that's cool. And the first time you stand up, that's cool. I never felt like I was learning to surf to be able to surf better in the future. Just enjoy where you're at. Enjoy the surfing itself and the speed and harmony, and the occasional seagull sitting in the water beside you!

ALISON: Every girl learns to surf differently. It took me three lessons to stand up, it took my sister sixteen seconds! I didn't have any flair for surfing but I have a lot of grit and determination, and that's got me farther than some people who were learning to surf at the same time as me who stood up immediately but don't practice—and that's okay too, not everybody wants to be out there every day. So don't compare yourself with others.

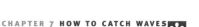

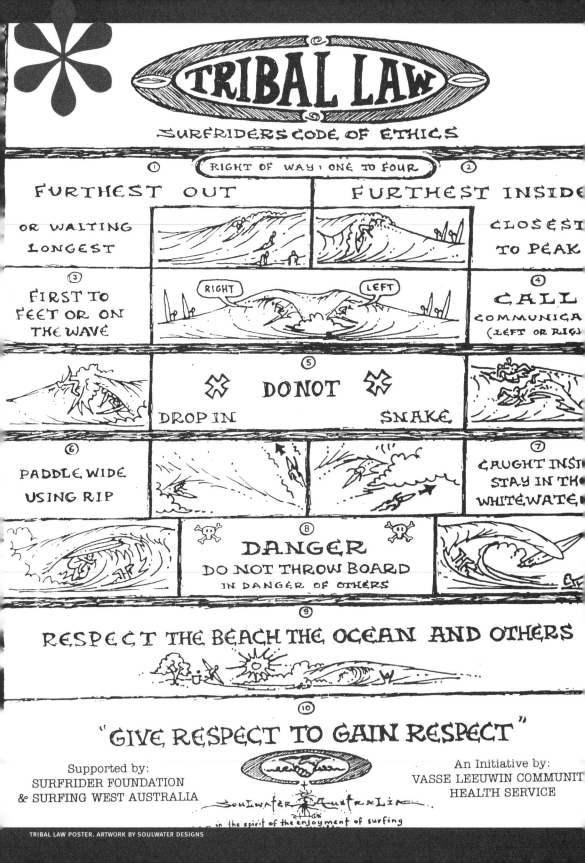

8

the*
rules

Learn:

Why **surfers** need rules. **Dropping in and how to avoid it; snaking; right-of-way when paddling out.** The gentle art of surf **conversation. Localism and how to handle it.**

Why do surfers need rules?

Whenever I meet people who don't surf, it reminds me how surfing looks from the outside: Surfers are all mellow, cruisey individuals who spend their time in the water waiting patiently for waves, watching the seagulls and fish, and chatting good-naturedly to one another about nothing in particular.

And it can be like that. It's just that more often it's like this: Paddle out, and you get the feeling that all the other surfers are thinking the same thing—one more surfer in the water means fewer waves for the rest of us. You smile at someone; they turn away. You paddle for a wave; another surfer drops in on you. When you paddle back out, someone almost runs you over. By the time you're ready for your second wave, you're feeling more stressed than if you'd just spent the last fifteen minutes in peak-hour traffic. What's going on here?

It's ironic that surfers often turn to the ocean environment for a bit of stress relief only to find, on getting out there, that it's just as stressful as life on land. With more surfers in the water now than ever before, surf breaks all over the world are more crowded and surfing, particularly at city beaches, is more competitive. As one of my friends once said, "Surfing is the only sport where you have to compete when you're training." It can also be more of a social experience—in that you're interacting with other people a lot of the time—than a natural one. For all these reasons, we need rules so everyone out there is on the same page when it comes to knowing where they should be and who they need to give way to.

Rules to surf by

Back in the old days, surfers learned the rules in a kind of organic way. Whoever taught you to surf, usually your "old man" or your brother (women surfers were few and far between), passed them on to you or you learned by trial and error: that is, by making mistakes and getting yelled at, preferably by your friends.

These days it's only marginally more organized. With the exception of a few Surfer's Code plaques dotted around the world (see box on page 152), the rules aren't really written down anywhere. Surf schools teach basic right-of-way, but a two-hour lesson isn't long enough to introduce you to all the situations you might encounter. The rules aren't even really enforced, unless you count the scorn and abuse you might attract if you break one.

Instead, right-of-way rules are just passed on from experienced

THE TRIBE HAS SPOKEN . . .

Back in 1996, surfing legends Nat Young and Robert Conneeley, along with long-time Australian surfer Peter Cuming and surfing artist Rosco Kermode, came up with the idea of installing weatherproof plaques explaining the rules of surfing at designated surf spots around Australia. The plaques were installed at Margaret River, Western Australia's premier surf spot, and at several spots around Byron Bay, on the east coast. In 2003 the famous Bells Beach surfing community created a series of Spirit of Surfing stones to urge surfers to respect the ocean, the land, and one another. More recently, Nat Young has been working with surfing elders all over the globe to develop an internationally recognizable surfing code of ethics. Now, Malibu Beach and Ventura County, California, are expressing interest in installing the new Surfer's Code plaques, and other surf

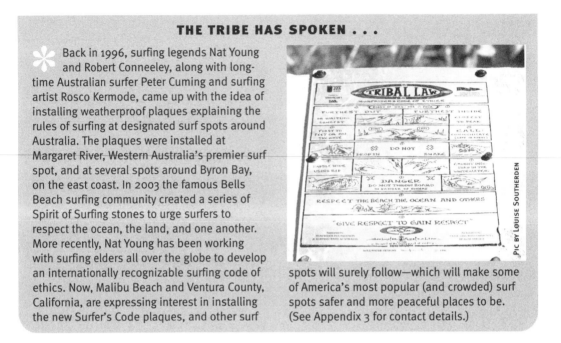

PIC BY LOUISE SOUTHERDEN

spots will surely follow—which will make some of America's most popular (and crowded) surf spots safer and more peaceful places to be. (See Appendix 3 for contact details.)

surfers to novices as a kind of code of ethics that surfers implicitly agree to abide by, on the whole, for the sake of safety and sanity in the surf. Whether or not you learn them is up to you, but they're as important as knowing how to paddle out and stand up on your board.

Dropping in

Once upon a time, surfboards weren't designed to go along the wave in one direction or the other; when you caught a wave, you headed straight for the beach, which meant that sharing waves wasn't a problem. It was almost a case of the more the merrier—ever seen one of those old surf movies where ten surfers are standing shoulder to shoulder, riding a wave together, everyone having the time of their lives?

With advances in surfboard design in the late 1950s, surfers started getting the crazy idea that it was more fun to trim along a wave than to go straight ahead, and the "one surfer per wave" concept came into being. Suddenly it became critical to have a rule to let everyone know who had the right-of-way.

So surfing got its first and most important rule: The surfer closest to the breaking part of the wave has the right-of-way. If another surfer cuts in, in front of the first surfer, she is "dropping

*tip

Just to confuse matters, "drop in" also means "takeoff," as in "Did you see me drop into that set wave?"

in." It goes like this: there are two surfers, Lucy and Zoe. Lucy takes off on a wave. Almost immediately, Zoe takes off in front of her. According to the "don't drop in" rule, which is pretty universal, it was Lucy's wave. In other words, Zoe dropped in on Lucy. Or, in still other words, Lucy was on the inside and Zoe was on the outside, so it was Lucy's wave.

If you only remember one rule when you're out in the surf, make sure it's this one: don't drop in. In case you're wondering, it's bad to drop in because:

- It spoils the wave for the surfer who has the right-of-way—if you drop in on someone, not only are you in their way, but you force the open face of the wave to crumble and break in front of them, prematurely ending their ride.
- It's dangerous, or can be—two surfers riding a wave in close proximity, even when they both know what they're doing, can have serious consequences in a wipeout, with *two* surfboards getting tossed around in the whitewater, *two* sets of fins, *two* leashes to get tangled . . . you get the picture.
- It's widely regarded as disrespectful and selfish—accidents can be forgiven but intentional dropping in is basically like saying, "I don't care about anyone else, I'm here to ride as many waves as I can."

To avoid dropping in on someone

Always glance back over your shoulder when you paddle for a wave in a crowded lineup; if you see someone else taking off or riding the wave you're going for, stop paddling for it. Also, and this is more common courtesy than part of the "don't drop in" rule, if

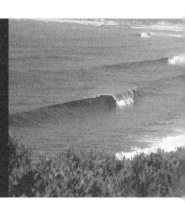

LOATA: It's important to be aware of the people around you, because sometimes you're so focused, like "I'm on the wave!," and you don't realize that someone else has the right-of-way to the right or left of you. I sat down with a friend and asked about the code of conduct in the surf because I didn't want to go out there and get yelled at and be oblivious . . . so when I go out now, I see where everyone is. Now I do it subconsciously but when you're new, you've got to be alert, like, "Okay, everyone's over there so where do I place myself?" It's a lot more involved than just paddling out there.

you see someone on the inside just *paddling* for the wave you wanted, give them the benefit of the doubt; assume they're going to catch that wave, and let them have it. You never know when you might want others to do the same for you.

What if I (accidentally!) drop in on someone?

If you've already caught the wave, try to get off it as soon as you can to give the other surfer (you know, the one surfing behind you!) the rest of the ride at least. This can be tricky, though: flicking off the wave requires some board control, and falling or jumping off your board can cause it to spear into the other surfer. Your best bet is to ride the wave safely to the shoulder and turn off as best you can. Don't forget to say "Sorry." More often than not, the surfer you dropped in on won't mind—accidents happen, and other surfers tend to be more forgiving when you're female.

What if someone drops in on me?

It's a fact of surfing life that sooner or later someone is going to drop in on you. How you handle it is up to you, but there are a couple of ways to keep your cool and make sure it doesn't happen again (that day anyway):

- When you're paddling for a wave and someone ahead of you looks like they're paddling for the same wave, let them know you're there: a single "Yep!" is often enough.

- Call "Left!" or "Right!"; many drop-ins occur because the dropper-inner isn't sure which way the other surfer is going to go on the wave.

- If they keep going and actually do drop in on you, you have a right to call them off your wave: yelling "Oi!" is an old Aussie favorite, but any shout will do. Hopefully they'll get the message; otherwise you can assume they know you're there but don't care that they broke the cardinal rule. Beyond that, there's not much you can do until you paddle back out—then you might want to say something to let them know that dropping in on you is *not* okay.

- Give everyone at least two chances: Assume the first drop-in is an accident. If they do it again, have a word with them.

There is one more way to avoid being dropped in on: show you can surf. When you're learning, you're particularly vulnerable to drop-ins because other surfers will assume you're not going to make the takeoff—that is, they'll think you're going to wipe out pretty early in the ride and assume that they may as well go for the wave themselves. Some surfers see it as their civic duty to not let a single wave go unridden!

The best way to deal with this attitude is by honing your skills and showing that you can ride every wave you paddle for—maybe not as they would ride it, but at least well enough to ensure the wave wasn't wasted. It can be stressful having to prove yourself every time you paddle out, but the incentive is that the better you surf, the more waves you'll get.

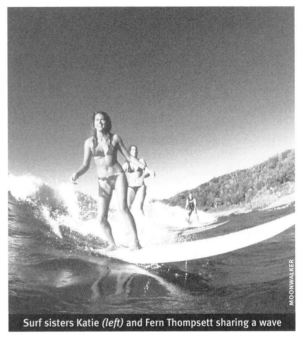

Surf sisters Katie *(left)* and Fern Thompsett sharing a wave

Is dropping in ever okay?

When you're surfing with friends, or if someone gives you permission to drop in on them—for example, they've seen how long you've been waiting for a wave and have taken pity on you, and, even though they want to catch the next wave themselves, they're prepared to share (who said chivalry was dead?)—then it's okay to drop in. Sometimes the surfer on the inside will be too deep (too close to the breaking part of the wave) to make it out onto the clean wave face; if you see the wave closing out in front of them, it's okay to "drop in" (in fact, it's technically not a drop-in, because the other surfer will probably be under a truckload of whitewater by the time you catch the wave).

Whose wave is it anyway? (Other right-of-way rules)

Besides "don't drop in," there are a couple of other rules for determining who has the right-of-way when two surfers are going for the same wave:

✳ tip

Surfing crowded breaks can be demoralizing if you're not catching waves, so surf at uncrowded breaks whenever you can. Head up or down the coast to remote beach breaks, surf early, or surf a second-rate peak where you're sure to get more waves than on the best and most crowded peak.

Farther out or waiting longer. When two surfers are on the same wave but neither is closer to the curl than the other, the surfer who is farther from the beach or has been waiting longer has the right-of-way. This rule is not often adhered to in crowded city lineups.

First to their feet or first on the wave. When two surfers on the same wave are riding different craft, the rules get a bit fuzzy (see below).

The long and the short of it

Both these rules can add fuel to the longboard–shortboard fire that was lit when shortboards were invented back in the late sixties. All other differences aside, there is one indisputable fact: longboard-ers, by virtue of their longer, more buoyant boards, can catch waves earlier, and therefore farther out, than shortboarders (who have to wait for waves to be steeper and closer to shore before they can catch them).

So a shortboarder might be paddling for a wave that a long-boarder has already caught, and even though neither of them is on the inside of the other, the longboarder will have right-of-way because she got to her feet and got onto the wave first. This is one reason there can be tension between longboarders and short-boarders—longboarders can potentially hog the waves because they can take advantage of this "first on the wave" rule. Most beginners' surfboards are classed as longboards so you'll have this advantage; don't abuse the privilege. A little wave-sharing goes a long way toward goodwill between surfers of all craft.

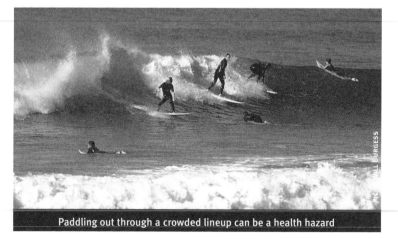
Paddling out through a crowded lineup can be a health hazard

No snaking

If you see a wave coming and paddle to the inside of a surfer who would have caught it if you hadn't been there, it's called "snaking." It's almost as low as dropping in and even harder to enforce because it's so sneaky: When it's crowded, it's hard to tell the difference between honest-to-goodness paddling into position and snaking. It really depends on the surfer's attitude and how aware she is of other surfers. Right-of-way in this case is about showing a little consideration. If you've just had a wave and someone else gets a chance for one, let her take it. Waves are like buses: If you miss one, there'll be another one along shortly.

"Right-of-way" when you're paddling out

It's more difficult to know who has right-of-way when you're paddling out, but there are guidelines. Sure, it's probably the responsibility of the surfer riding the wave to avoid obstacles (like surfers paddling out) in her path, but in the interests of your own safety, try to keep out of the way of surfers riding waves.

In other words, there are a few things you can do when you're paddling out (more out of a sense of self-preservation than because it's law) to make sure you don't get in the way of the surfers riding the oncoming waves:

● Paddle wide of the break if you can. That is, try not to paddle straight back out through the surf zone where you're likely to encounter surfers riding waves head on (let's hope not literally!). This is not always possible at beach breaks, where you have to paddle back through the waves to get out, and that's when the following rules kick in:

● Stay in the whitewater. If there's a wave coming and you think you can paddle over the shoulder, in front of the surfer riding the wave (so you don't have to duck-dive or turtle-roll), don't. Hold your course and paddle behind the surfer—even if it means getting thrashed by the whitewater.

● Don't throw your board if there's a chance it might hit someone. Remember the bit about bailing your board in Chapter 6? The same principles apply here. You might have checked behind you before you threw your board and dived for safety, but sometimes your lone board can hit the surfer riding the wave you just dived under.

Talking the talk—the gentle art of surf conversation

"What do you talk about out there?" one of my non-surfing friends asked me the other day. It took me a while to realize why I found it hard to answer: Most of the time surfers don't talk much when they're in the water. Sure, you might swap information about the waves or weather, ask what time is low tide, or comment on someone's great ride; surfers who know each other will be more chatty; and sometimes you might start talking to someone sitting near you, just to be friendly. But mostly it's pretty quiet out there—and that's the way most surfers like it. For many of us, surfing is a time to chill out, be alone with our thoughts and have nothing to do but catch the next wave.

You talkin' to me?

One of the great things about surfing, particularly when you want a bit of solitude, is that it's perfectly acceptable not to talk while you're out in the water. Not only that, but if you are talking to someone and, midconversation, midsentence, or even midword, a wave comes your way, no one expects you to do anything more than turn your board around and catch it—the assumption being that you'll resume the conversation (or not) when you've paddled back out. The unspoken rule is: We're here to surf; talking is just something to do while we're waiting for the next wave, and if you want to sit in silence, staring at the horizon, that's okay too.

The dating game

You might come across this little scenario sometime in your surfing life. You're sitting in the lineup quietly minding your own business, when some guy paddles over and starts chatting to you. That's all very well if his intention is just to be friendly and you're as interested as he seems to be, but what if he has a not-so-hidden agenda and before long you're fending off pickup lines? Or, worse, he starts showing off his latest moves to impress you. This is uncool. We're all surfers out there, and female surfers in particular have struggled to at least lower the barriers between males and females out in the water; as soon as a guy decides to hit on you, those barriers are back up again.

How to handle this? Don't be rude but tell him straight: You're just out there to surf. If Mr. Wrong persists, paddle away. Be clear about your boundaries; your needs are as important as anyone else's. Besides, it's not your responsibility to entertain him while he's waiting for his next wave.

Then there are guys who won't talk to you in case you *think* they're hitting on you. That's when being the only girl in the water can be a lonely experience. Older surfers don't seem to worry about this so much, so they can be the most approachable if you want some company out there.

Less (talk) is more (waves)

There's another reason surfers often don't talk much in the water: it's distracting. Anything but a light 'n' easy conversation can take your attention away from what the waves are doing and how the conditions might be changing. When you realize that you—and probably the person you're talking to—aren't catching as many waves as you'd like, it might be time to take a break. You can even be open about it: "Hey, we'd better stop talking and start surfing!"

There is, however, one time when surfers *love* talking: when they scored perfect waves earlier that day or week. "You shoulda been here yesterday/last week/an hour ago," they say. Seriously, though, swapping stories when you're back on the beach about great waves (and wipeouts!) is a fine way to bond with your fellow surfers.

To share or not to share—the surfer's eternal struggle

There are two occasions when surfers raise their voices: to get you off a wave they've claimed as theirs (see Dropping In on pages 152–7) and to "hoot" you when you're paddling for a good wave or riding one. They kind of cancel each other out, but that's

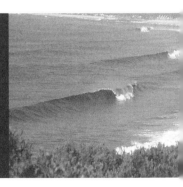

ALISON: I think as women we're very lucky to have this extra ability to read emotions. And simply because someone looks scary, it doesn't always mean they are. I was surfing at Manly Beach [in Sydney] a few months ago and there was a really scary-looking bloke and he wasn't talking to anybody, he had a kind of menacing aura. Then these dolphins came by and he said, "Look at the dolphins!" He had this big grin on his face and we ended up having a nice chat. So I think it's too easy to scare yourself into not going out. Feel it out when you get out there.

the nature of surfing: Surfers are constantly torn between a share-the-waves ideal (where you get as much joy from someone else riding a wave as riding one yourself) and making the most of your time in the water by catching as many waves as you can. At the end of the day, surfing's not a team sport, but it can be a shared experience. It all comes down to the attitude you take out there with you.

Locals only

Surfers are territorial creatures. Although traveling for waves is an essential part of the surfing life if you want to progress in your surfing, there's something about surfing your local break and getting to know it like an old friend that is close to every surfer's heart. It's almost as if it becomes an extension of your domain, your backyard, a place where you know everyone in the lineup, as well as where to paddle out, where to take off, and how to surf the waves.

The downside of this familiarity—for visiting surfers anyway—is the potential for locals to dominate a surf spot in a way that makes it unpleasant for anyone else to surf there. That's localism: when surfers who live and/or surf at the spot in question think that because they're locals they have right-of-way on every wave there. (Most surfers don't subscribe to this narrow approach—not just out of common decency, but because they know that, sooner or later, they too will want to travel for waves and no one can be a local everywhere.)

At its most benign, localism expresses itself as Locals Only graffiti spray-painted at the parking lot or on the walls near the break. Or local surfers will snake and drop in on visiting surfers, or deliberately aim their boards at non-locals in the lineup when they're on a wave. More extreme cases can involve surf rage (fights in the water or on the beach) or vandalism against your property, mostly the car that brought you there (there's a kind of symbolism in that), such as rubbing wax on your windshield (very hard to remove), breaking into your car, or slashing your tires.

The bottom line is that localism is rooted in fear: fear that their break will become overcrowded if too many more surfers start surfing there—which translates to fewer waves for those who try to claim ownership over that which can't be owned.

Who are the locals anyway?

The definition of "local" at any given beach is fuzzy at the best of times: locals can be those surfers who live within walking distance, those who surf there every day (but might not live there), or those who have been surfing there longer than anyone else. The best approach when you paddle out somewhere you've never surfed before is to assume that most of the other surfers are locals—and therefore deserve some respect. Before long you'll be able to distinguish the surfers who seem to know the break from those who look like they've never surfed there before either.

How to survive localism

Be mentally prepared. It's not always easy to anticipate where "heavy" (intimidating) locals will be. Sometimes it's in remote breaks that don't get many visitors. Sometimes city surf beaches will be just as locally dominated—particularly when there's a good swell. When the takeoff spot is small or crowded, or the waves are heavy, that's when you have to be especially aware of other surfers, locals or not.

- Whenever you surf a new spot, respect the surfers out there who look like they know what they're doing and know other surfers in the lineup. This means giving them plenty of space— if they look like they're taking a wave, give them the benefit of the doubt and don't drop in.

- Know your place in the pecking order. The rules aren't just about right-of-way, they're about consideration and respect for your fellow surfers. So when you paddle back out after catching a wave, don't paddle straight back to the inside position ready for your next ride. There's a lot to be said for knowing your place in the pecking order and waiting your turn.

- Obey the rules even more strictly when you're surfing a new spot than you would anywhere else.

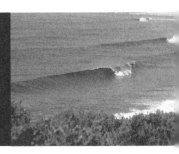

ALISON: My surfing philosophy is: Have fun, don't hurt anybody. And just because someone's not riding the board that you prefer, it doesn't mean they're a kook or an idiot. Just because someone's on a bodyboard, don't call them a shark biscuit or a speed hump. We all know how bad it feels to be put down by somebody, so I don't think we should be carrying that vibe. I think women are smart enough to be over that boys' club stuff.

When you're a local

Sooner or later, if you start surfing one area more than any other, you might become a local yourself. Wield your power generously. By being a local, you're going to understand the break better than visiting surfers and therefore catch more waves legitimately anyway, so there's no need to steal waves from other surfers. Do your bit for world peace: Smile at a non-local!

Last words

R-E-S-P-E-C-T. As with any kind of etiquette, the bottom line is respect: so if you don't know the rules, just try to be considerate of other surfers and beach-users. This extends to the natural environment as well. Because people often respect surfers for being able to ride waves and understand the ocean, they often follow our example. If we respect the beach, the ocean, and one another, other people might too.

Smile. It's a fact of life that when you paddle out into the surf, most surfers will regard you, at least initially, as their enemy. If you smile and acknowledge other surfers when you get out the back, it'll let them know you're aware of them and that you're not just out there for yourself. You might be pleasantly surprised to find they're not as unfriendly as you first thought.

Girl power. Although equality rules in the surf, sometimes being a female has advantages. Most guy surfers regard dropping in on girl surfers as a pretty low act—in fact, most guys will call you onto waves, not try to steal them from you. As for localism, females in

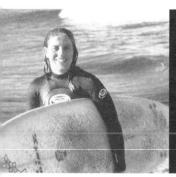

ESTHER: Because I started surfing late—I was in my twenties and I'm thirty-one now—when I go in the water, there's a lot of guys who have been surfing since they were very young so they can surf so much better than me. So I have to tell myself, This is my place too, I can have fun here and I can be here, and I'm enjoying it so I'll keep doing it. It's better to look at them and think, It's cool what they're doing, than to be intimidated by them and feel that you're not supposed to be out there.

the surf are often seen as less of a threat than male surfers; call it sexist, but if it saves your car tires, be thankful! Many guys even welcome more girls into the lineup, claiming that our presence eases the testosterone-charged atmosphere and creates a more relaxed vibe out there.

BYO peace. People's lives often follow them out into the lineup: if they're having a tough time at home or work, it can show in their surfing or the way they act in the water. It's easy to react to this attitude with more aggression, and as women we're probably more sensitive to the social environment—the vibe—out in the lineup than many of our male counterparts. Step back from it and try not to take it personally; it's probably not about you anyway.

Know your place. No matter how other people treat you, it's handy to remember that you have as much right to be out there in the water as anyone else.

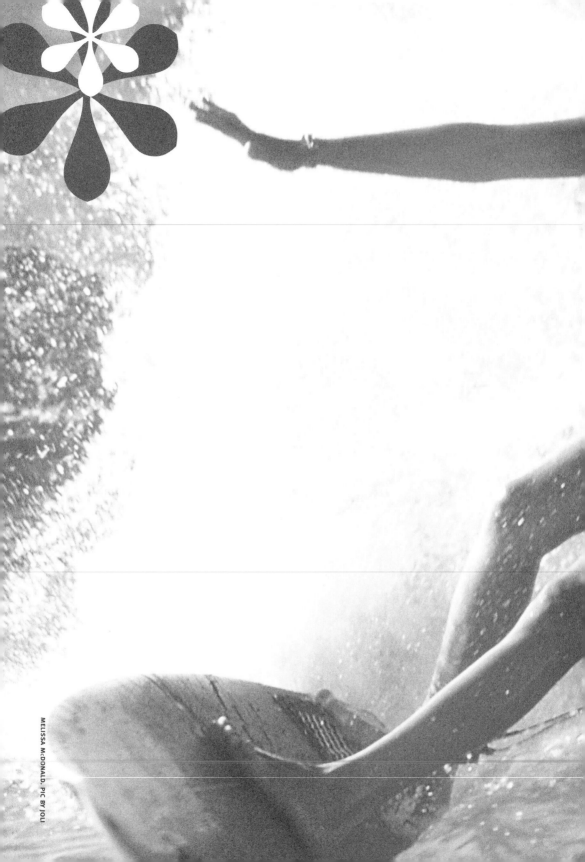

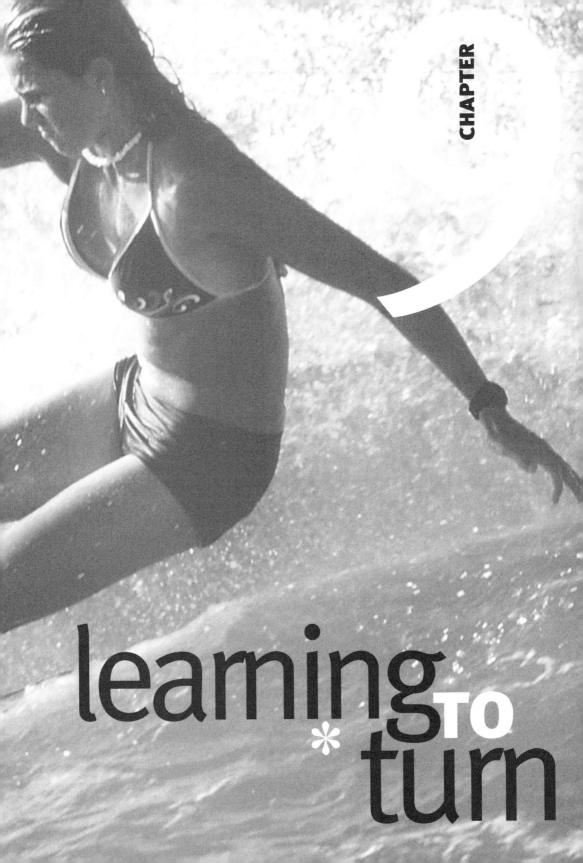

learning *to turn

Learn:

What to do after you can stand up on your board—surfing **straight** to the beach, **riding** along the face of the wave, and turning. **About wave shape: rights, lefts, closeouts, and peeling waves.** How to do **S-turns,** the prelude to real turning. **How to do frontside and backside bottom turns.** Ten steps to turning your **board. How to surf with style.** How to get **off** the wave.

*

You've been waiting for just the right wave, sitting patiently on your board watching the approaching bumps and trying to pick one that (a) won't break on top of you and (b) you can catch. At last, here it comes, *your* wave. You paddle for it, glancing over your shoulder now and then to keep an eye on its progress and make sure you're in the right spot for the takeoff. Paddle, paddle, the back of your board lifts and you've got it! You spring to your feet in one smooth movement. You're up. What now?

Once you're comfortable standing up for more than a few seconds, it's time to start steering your board across the face of that glassy green wave.

Back to the whitewater

But first . . . I know it seems like a backward step to go back to the whitewater yet again, but I can assure you it's a necessary one. Remember when you were doing the tummy-surfing thing? When you leaned left and then right as you rode the whitewater to the beach, to get a feel for how your board would respond to your movements? It's time to take that board knowledge a step further.

The weighting game

The first thing to practice is transferring your weight: to your back foot, to your front foot, and back again. You don't have to move your feet, just lean your upper body over your back knee and then over your front knee. You don't even have to think about where you want to go at this stage, just let your movements determine where the board goes.

You can also try putting your weight on your heels, then your toes, and see what your board does. I don't want to spoil the surprise, but basically, when you put weight onto your toes, your board starts to turn the way you're facing; when you lean onto your heels, your board will turn away from the way you're facing.

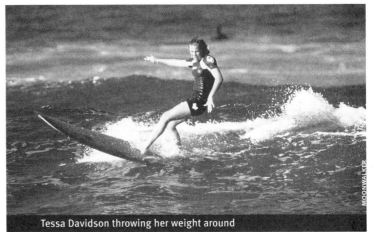

Tessa Davidson throwing her weight around

MOONWALKER

Going for green (waves, that is)

When you get used to how your board behaves as you move your weight around, you can take these lessons into the green waves. The beauty of surfing unbroken waves is that, unlike the whitewater, you now have somewhere to go: along the clear, unblemished face of the wave. Traveling across the face of the wave is where it's all at.

Straight ahead, driver!

When you first start surfing green waves, you'll probably feel most comfortable aiming your board straight for the beach—just as you did in the whitewater. This is a good way to get a feel for the drop and get comfortable with the whole timing thing: that is, standing up just as the wave is breaking.

What you'll probably notice is that when you aim straight for the beach on a green wave, the wave will break around you or onto the tail of your board, and you'll end up surfing in the whitewater again anyway. D'oh! It's a good exercise to show you how waves behave and motivate you for the next step: going across the wave.

Surfing across the wave

When you're comfortable surfing straight, it's time to try gliding across the wave in the direction it's breaking. It's just like traversing on your snowboard, except the "mountains" are a lot smaller and they move! The aim of the game is to steer your board *away* from the breaking part of the wave and *toward* the shoulder, the open part of the wave. So if a wave breaks to the right, ride it to the right; vice versa for left-breaking waves.

A word about wave shape

The tricky part about this is that not every wave will allow you to surf across it. You can't surf along a wave that has no open wall, no matter how perfect the conditions are. This is where two of the most important skills you will ever learn come in: wave selection (choosing which wave to catch) and reading the wave when you're up and riding it. The more time you put into actually looking at waves, the more your surfing will progress.

Most waves fall somewhere between two extremes: closeouts and peeling waves.

- A closeout is a wave that breaks simultaneously along its entire length. Closeouts (swimmers call them "dumpers") aren't very popular with surfers because there's nowhere to go when you catch them. Catching closeouts is a great way to practice your takeoffs though—they can break quickly and there's no time to do anything else!

- Peeling waves, on the other hand, offer a whole lot more. Because they break along their length, like a zipper closing, staying ahead of the breaking part means you've got a nice open wall to ride. Peeling waves break either to the right or to the left.

✳tip

Watching other surfers doesn't just help you learn to surf, it tells you how the waves are breaking. When you're sitting out the back, watch other surfers take off. Are they going right or left? Are they getting long rides, or are they getting caught by the breaking part of the wave almost as soon as they stand up?

If only it were this simple! The fact is, waves are unpredictable creatures (okay, they're not really creatures, but you may come to think of them that way when you've been out in the sun too long). You might arrive at the beach, only to find every wave is a close-out—which means it's time to head for another beach—or you might find that every wave is a perfect peeler. Or the waves peel for a while and then close out, or get slower or steeper; the variations are endless. This is one of the reasons surfers seek out point breaks and reef breaks, where the waves break the same way every time—you can relax a bit in the knowledge that there won't be too many big surprises.

The more you surf, the better you will get at reading waves. Sometimes you'll be caught out—for example, you might be high on a wave and it will suddenly get steep and break, leaving you nowhere to go but down and out.

Start facing the wave

You'll soon notice that because you stand sideways on your board with one foot in front of the other, some waves will be easier to ride than others. Most surfers find it easier to surf on their "frontside" (facing the wave) than on their "backside" (with their back to the wave they're riding).

This is because when you're surfing on your frontside, you can see the wave you're about to surf across, you can see if it's going to shut down (another term for "close out") up ahead and, as you lean forward for balance, you're also leaning into the wave, so it feels more stable.

When you're surfing backside, with your back to the wave, it's a little trickier. Because the wave is behind you, you have to twist around to look over your leading shoulder to see what the wave's doing; this can cause you to lean back, which feels awkward at first. Of course, you'll need to learn to surf this way sooner or later,

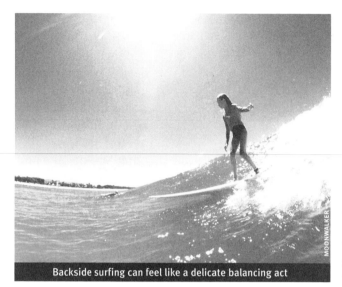

Backside surfing can feel like a delicate balancing act

but it may as well be later, after you've got your confidence from surfing frontside.

So when you're getting used to surfing across the wave, try to surf facing the wave. It's not a matter of changing your stance to make it easier (unless you're Kelly Slater, who seems to be able to surf either way—called "switch-foot"—with ease), it's a matter of choosing the waves that allow you to surf on your frontside.

All you have to remember is this: **If you're a regular footer, go right** (that is, try to catch waves that break to the right). **If you're a goofyfoot, go left.**

S-turns

Remember when you were back in the whitewater, transferring your weight onto your front foot and your back foot? It's time to apply that lesson to green waves, so you can start zigzagging and doing gentle S-turns up and down the face of the wave as you ride across it. This is a natural stopover between just going across the wave, and your ultimate destination: doing full turns. Oh, and it's fun!

Teaching someone how to turn their surfboard is a bit like teaching someone how to dance. You can teach them the moves, but you can't teach them how to feel the wave and tune in to its rhythm. The more you surf, the more you develop an intuitive

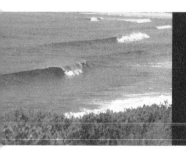

LOATA: I learned on my backhand [backside], for some reason, even though I was goofy. I think I always imagined surfing to be so hard I just thought that's how you surf, with your back to the wave. And people would say, "No, no, no, you've got to *face* the wave, that's the most natural way." Once I started doing that, I thought, This is so much easier than what I was doing!

feeling for your surfboard and for each wave you ride, which will help you more than any rigid set of instructions.

Having said that, here are a few tips:

Lean and twist. As you become more comfortable with the way your board moves, how much pressure you need on your back foot to make it change direction, and how it speeds up when you lean forward, you can try making a few more movements, like twisting your upper body to the right when you want your board to go right, and twisting to the left to go left. Notice, too, how the pressure changes on your toes and heels as you veer right and left.

The middle way. Lean too far back, and you'll fall off the back of your board. But if you don't lean far enough, your board won't turn at all. Like anything in life, it's about finding a balance. Also, the longer your board is, the more you will have to lean into your back foot to turn it. For boards over 9 foot, you actually have to walk up and down the board instead of just leaning.

Stay high. As you do your wiggly turns across the face of the wave, try to keep your board high up on the wave face. Not too high, or you can get caught by the lip and be unceremoniously dumped. And not too low in the trough part of the wave, or you'll lose speed and the breaking part of the wave will catch up with you and put an end to your fun. The aim is to keep your board moving.

Don't be ambitious. At this point, it's not important how many turns you do on each wave. Doing S-turns is about feeling the wave and the board under your feet. Every wave is different anyway; some will give you room to fit in lots of turns; others will end before they've even begun.

Doing wiggly turns across the face of the wave is a great way to get ready for doing proper turns, because it gets you used to balancing on a surfboard as it changes direction (even slightly), and it lets you explore different parts of the wave without committing to doing full turns. One thing you might notice is that your board picks up speed as you ride down the face of the wave—even on small waves, it's like taking off all over again!—and loses speed as you go up the face of the wave. This is an important lesson. When you start linking turns, you'll need to use the speed you pick up coming *down* the wave to propel you back *up* toward the top of the wave.

Why turn?

Once you're comfortable zigzagging up and down the face of the wave, it's time to try steering your board through a real turn—that is, a turn where you actually change direction on the wave.

This is a big step. Until now, all you had to do was ride the darn thing; now you've got to control its movements! In fact, you might even be asking yourself why you need to bother turning your board when cruising along the face of the wave is so much fun. Well, there are a few good reasons:

● **Safety.** Being able to maneuver your surfboard, even slightly, stops surfing from becoming a contact sport. It's your duty as a surfer to learn how to turn your board, despite what one of my (male) friends once said to me, "You don't need to turn a mini-longboard (a beginners' board), you just need to wave your arms around and say, 'Get out of the way, get out of the way!' "

● **Speed.** Turning helps you to maintain and generate speed by moving you through different parts of the wave. It also puts you in control of your craft; without turning, you're just another piece of flotsam washing in from the ocean.

● **Sensations.** Nothing beats those delicious G-forces you get when you do a nice carving turn. It's what surfing is all about.

● **Self-expression.** Like the clothes you wear, the way you walk, or how you speak, turning your surfboard allows you to express who you are in the water. This is good news when you're starting out because it means there's no right or wrong way to surf. Surfing is the ultimate free-form activity.

Surfing in the pocket

There is one more vitally important reason for turning: to stay where the wave's energy is most intense, usually just in front of the breaking part of the wave, a place called the "pocket." Surfing in the pocket is what makes the difference between a great ride and an average ride, and turning your board is how you stay there.

On most waves, if you don't turn your board, you'll be carried full steam ahead onto the shoulder, the weakest part of the wave, where you risk coming to a complete standstill unless the wave overtakes you—either way, your glorious ride is over. Being able to turn your board means that when you sense yourself getting too far ahead of the breaking part of the wave, you can turn back into the pocket. It's hard to describe how it feels to be "locked in" or surfing in "perfect trim." It's like being in love: you just know.

Move that body

If you thought paddling gave you a workout, try turning your surfboard. Every part of your body has a role to play when you start doing turns.

Feet first. Your feet are the two most important players in turning your board. Make sure they're not too close together—they should be about three feet apart for stability. And not too far back—you don't want to fall off the back of the board. According to surf coach Priscilla-Anne Hensler, your front foot is your accelerator and your back foot is your brake. "When the wave slows down, put as much weight as you can onto your front foot and drive the board for acceleration. When the wave's really steep or really fast, you may want to put on your brake a little bit. . . . Sometimes beginners get up and they've got all their weight on their back foot and they're going nowhere. And I say to them, 'Lean onto your front foot—accelerate, accelerate!' And the next thing you know they're shooting toward the beach!"

Stay low. Keep your center of gravity low by bending your knees (it gives your thighs a workout!). Your legs are the quiet achievers of surfing.

Do the twist. Twist your upper body like a spring—when it untwists, you'll get a release of energy that will propel you through your turn. Point to where you want to go with your front hand—this will turn your shoulders to face the direction you want to go—and follow through with your body.

The eyes have it. Your eyes are your steering wheels—where they go, you go. So when you're turning, look to where you want to go next.

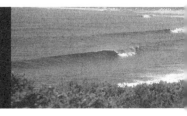

Turning your board

The difference between S-turns and full turns is really just a matter of degree, a matter of extending each S so that your board actually changes direction. You do this by making stronger, more defined movements; the more you move, the more your board moves. This requires a bit more balance and coordination—you're more likely to fall off when doing a turn that takes your board through 180 degrees than a turn that makes your board's nose wiggle from right to left. But where the risks are greater, so are the rewards—there's nothing like successfully pulling off your first "real" turn.

Where to start

When you take off on a wave, you've got two choices in terms of when you can start turning your board. The decision-making point comes when you start paddling for the wave:

● You can paddle onto the wave at an angle, which means that, as soon as you get to your feet, your board is already heading across the wave in the direction you want to go. All you have to do then is keep up your speed by doing turns as you cruise along the face of the wave. This is an easy place to start, because you don't have to turn your board so radically at the critical bottom part of the wave face. It's also handy when the waves are steep, to avoid nose-diving.

● You can aim your board straight to the beach, which means that, as you stand up, your board will go directly down the face of the wave (you literally "take the drop"), and when you reach the bottom, you'll have to do a turn (called a "bottom turn") so you can start riding the wave to the right or the left. The main advantage of doing this is that it's exciting!

The bottom turn

This is the very first turn that everyone learns to do, mainly because it's the first turn you do on a wave, but also because it sets you up for your entire ride. A strong bottom turn allows you to use the speed from your takeoff to go along the wave or up toward the lip in preparation for your next turn, which will probably be a "top turn" (the turn you do at the top of the wave). The bottom turn is also the foundation for every other maneuver you'll do on a wave (cutbacks, re-entries, and so on).

EMY: When you're learning how to catch a ball, you've got to keep your eye on the ball. It's the same when you're surfing, you've got to keep your eye on the wave that's forming in front of you so you can see where you're going to go.

Frontside bottom turns

It's a good idea to start on your frontside again, just as you did when you were learning to go across the face of the wave. That is, start practicing frontside bottom turns and, when you feel comfortable with those, progress to backside bottom turns.

A frontside bottom turn will make you turn to the right if you're a regular footer, and to the left if you're goofy. Let's go through it as if you're a regular footer, riding a right-hander:

1. Paddle onto the wave with your board angling to the right and stand up in one smooth movement before you get to the bottom of the wave.
2. Stay low and keep your weight over your back foot to stop your board from nose-diving. The more weight you put on your back foot, the more the nose of your board will lift out of the water, which makes your board less stable but easier to turn.
3. As you reach the bottom of the wave (it's probably a pretty small wave, so it won't take long), twist your shoulders slightly to the right so you're facing the wave (imagine you're pointing to two o'clock on an imaginary clock face on the deck of your board).
4. Lean into the face of the wave—on bigger waves, sticking your back hand into the face of the wave can help you to get your weight over; it also gives you a point around which to turn, kind of like planting a pole when you're skiing. You might feel your toes pressing into the board.
5. Take your eyes off the nose of your board and look where you want to go. It helps to point to where you want to go with your front arm as well.

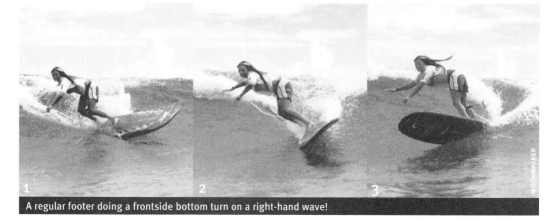

A regular footer doing a frontside bottom turn on a right-hand wave!

6. Your board starts to turn when your lower body—attached to your legs and therefore your board!—follows the example of your upper body and you find yourself untwisting and straightening up.

7. When you're about halfway through the turn and your board is starting to move up the face of the wave (it's now pointing away from the beach), move your weight forward a bit so that you drive the board around the pivot point at the tail of the board.

8. As you come out of the turn, move your weight over the center of your board so it's evenly distributed between both feet; then your board can gather speed by gliding across the surface of the wave. You can either go straight for a while or, when you get a bit more confident, go into a "top turn" (at the top of the wave).

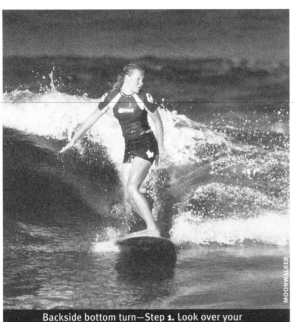

Backside bottom turn—Step **1.** Look over your leading shoulder

These steps are just a guideline. Turning is so intuitive that the best way to learn to turn is to get out in the water and play with it: see what happens when you move back and forward, lean, twist, shake, rattle, and roll. Oh, and be prepared to fall off—lots.

Backside bottom turns

Doing a bottom turn on your backside is the same as doing it on your frontside, with one major difference: you've got your back to the wave. Feels more awkward, huh? You can't see where you're going unless you swivel around; you can't see the wave and what it's going to do, which makes you feel more vulnerable. And it feels strange and different to be twisting your body this way. You'll probably fall off the first few times you try.

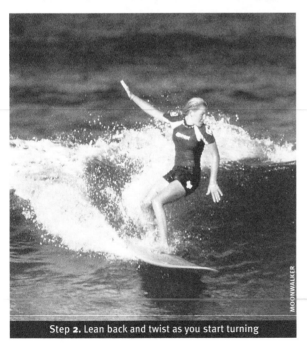

Step **2.** Lean back and twist as you start turning

No matter, just keep trying. Here's the drill:

1. Paddle onto the wave (it's a left this time, if you're a regular footer, as shown in the photos) and keep your weight on your back foot to stop yourself from nosediving. (See photos page 176)
2. Lean back into the heels of both feet. Your heels play a big part in your backside bottom turn—they allow you to get your weight onto that inside rail, the edge of your board around which you'll be turning.
3. Twist your upper body to the left— your left arm will be coming around behind you. Look over your left shoulder to where you want to go. If you've got the imaginary clock handy, you'll be pointing to ten o'clock with your leading arm.

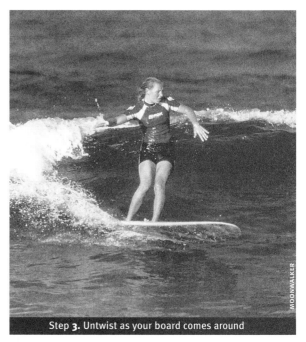

Step 3. Untwist as your board comes around

4. When you're about halfway through the turn, bring your weight forward over your front foot to steer your board around to the left.
5. As your body untwists, bring your weight into the center of your board. Voilà!

Short vs. long (boards, that is)

Longboards and shortboards turn differently, which is helpful to know if you're learning to surf on anything shorter than a mini-longboard.

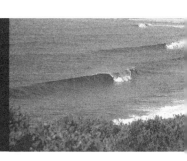

BEL: When you're doing a backside turn, just plonk your butt in the "lounge chair"—it's like sitting down in a lounge chair—to get the weight back into your heels. Don't stick your bottom out or you'll overbalance. You need to have your knees bent so that your center of gravity is low and you have less chance of falling off. So when you start to wobble on a wave, just drop—that'll stabilize you.

WHAT KIND OF SURFER ARE YOU?

According to a theory that's as old as surfing itself, there are two kinds of surfers. There are those who use the wave like a watery skate ramp, a liquid halfpipe, in order to do the maneuvers they want to do: launch themselves into airs, grind deep turns, snap their boards around. Then there are surfers whose maneuvers are dictated by the wave: the moves they perform are designed to keep them in the pocket, the most powerful spot in the wave, and by staying there they really ride the wave. Neither of these styles is better than the other; it's a matter of personal preference. They each have their place in the lineup.

Longboards (including mini-longboards) generally take more time to turn, which is why they're great for learning—there's more time to see what you're actually doing, and more time to correct it if you're not going where you want to go.

On a shortboard, you still have to keep your weight low, but you don't have to move around as much as you do on a longboard; as soon as you stand up, your back foot will already be over the fins and your front foot can stay where it is. You also use your rails (the edges of your board) more when turning a shortboard; whereas longboards pivot around the tail (which is why you need to get all your weight on your back foot for it to move). Shortboards are also more responsive—a slight shift in weight will make your board start turning—which is why they're not ideal for learning.

The learning-to-turn drill

To sum up, here are ten easy steps to learning how to turn your surfboard.

In the whitewater:

1. Tummy surfing. Practice catching broken waves—that is, the whitewater—and riding straight in to the beach while lying on your board.
2. Still lying on your board, grab your rails and lean to the left and right while you ride the whitewater, to see how moving your weight around on your board helps you to maneuver it.
3. Practice standing up on your board in the whitewater, and when you can stay on your feet for more than a few seconds, try transferring your weight onto your back foot (to slow down), then onto your front foot (to speed up), while heading straight to the beach.

In green waves:

4. Practice catching green waves and standing up as you drop down the face of the wave.
5. When you're confident enough to take off and stand for more than a few seconds, practice transferring your weight from your back foot to your front foot as you surf straight to the beach.
6. Ride across the wave, standing up, to the left or right; start on your frontside.
7. Do S-turns: combine going across the wave with transferring

your weight to your back foot, then your front foot, and see how your board zigzags or wiggles up and down the face of the wave.

8. Practice frontside bottom turns: that is, turning your board at the bottom of the wave and coming halfway up the face of the wave, while surfing on your frontside. Lean back, twist, then lean slightly forward, and look to where you want to go on the wave.

9. Practice backside bottom turns: same as above but while surfing on your backside. Lean into your heels, and look over your shoulder to where you want to go.

10. Paddle for a wave, stand up as you take the drop, and move your weight back to do a turn at the bottom of the wave. This will take you up the face of the wave about halfway, where you can traverse along the wave, do S-turns up and down the face of the wave, or do a top turn to take you back to the bottom of the wave. You're linking turns!

Connecting the dots

Once you know how to do frontside and backside bottom turns, you can try them out in all sorts of situations. Frontside bottom turns, for instance, aren't just good for turning at the bottom of the wave when you're surfing on your frontside. You can use them to escape closeouts: Imagine you're surfing along the wave on your backside when suddenly you realize the wave is going to dump in front of you; you do a frontside turn and behold! Now your board is aiming straight for the beach.

Or let's say you're surfing on your frontside and you want to turn away from the top of the wave and race down the face to pick up a bit of speed—that's when you can do a backside turn.

When you can turn your board both ways—to the right and to the left—you can try linking turns, so that you can change direction smoothly and efficiently. The end of one turn becomes the beginning of your next turn.

Elements of style

Linking turns takes you up the escalator and onto a whole new level in your surfing, one where you can start devel-

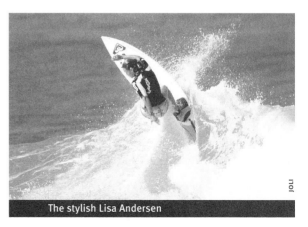

The stylish Lisa Andersen

oping your own surfing style. It'll probably be an unconscious thing at first, but the more confidence you develop, the more *you* will shine through in your surfing.

What makes a good surfing style? For me, it's when someone makes surfing look easy; she flows effortlessly with the wave and seems in tune with it. One of my favorite surfers is Lisa Andersen, because she surfs with such grace and power, and watching her surf makes me want to go surfing too.

There are no rights and wrongs when it comes to style, but it seems everyone has an opinion about what makes a good style:

Emy: Everyone has her own style, but if you just stay relaxed and fluid, you'll have no problems. If you're really tense or like a robot, you'll just fall off.

Loata: I like it when surfers use their bodies, their bodies are flexible. A good style is when it's like you're sitting in an invisible chair. A lot of longboarders are really graceful that way; there's no stress, it looks easy.

Deborah: I'm completely enamored of this girl I saw out in the water the other day at Malibu. It wasn't very warm, but she was in a bikini top and shorts, and she was riding a longboard. When she saw a wave coming, she paddled effortlessly toward it and then just stood up. She was so graceful. Before she hit the rocks, she gave the board a slight turn, stopped, and hopped right back into a sitting position. That's something I aspire to, that sort of grace in the water.

Exit stage left (or right)

There will be times when you need to get off the wave you're riding—quickly. Like when you've been surfing along its face and now, for no good reason, it's about to close out. Or it's getting a little too steep and you just want to get off. Or maybe it's been such a long ride that your legs are tired (it happens, particularly

SECTION, WHAT SECTION?

When an otherwise peeling wave breaks suddenly—closes out or shuts down—in front of you, that breaking part is called a "section," and unless you can get up enough speed to surf around the foam or do a maneuver over it, that's it, folks. As in:

Surfer A to Surfer B paddling back out after a wave: "How was that one?"

Surfer B: "It was a nice drop, but I didn't make it past the section."

on point breaks where the waves seem to go on forever!).

When you want to get off a wave, for whatever reason, there are a few options:

Straighten out. If you were going right, turn your board slightly to the left until you're aiming at the beach; vice versa for lefts. Besides jumping off your board midride, this is the easiest way to exit a wave. By straightening out, you'll usually shoot out in front of the wave. If you're not thrown off balance by the explosion of whitewater around you, you'll probably want to dive off your board as soon as you realize the ride's over: The longer your board keeps heading in to the beach, the farther you'll have to paddle back out.

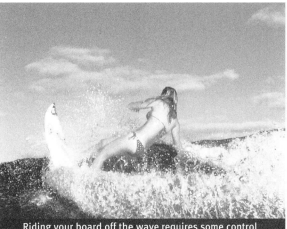
Riding your board off the wave requires some control

Ride your board off the wave before it shuts down. This is a bit trickier than straightening out because it requires more board control to aim for the fatter, shoulder part of the wave and ride out onto the flat water, where you can then lie down on your board and paddle back out. It's also more risky because, if you get caught at the top of a breaking wave, it can take you down and over the falls with it. But, if you pull it off, it saves struggling with the white-water and you won't lose your board, so you won't need to waste valuable paddling time getting back on it.

Kick out. Sometimes you and your board have to part company for there to be any chance of either of you surviving the breaking wave. That's when you need to know a couple of ways to "kick out" or escape a collapsing wave:

- Dive off your board and over the back of the wave, leaving your trusty board to deal with the consequences of the close-out. Because you and your board are going to be heading in opposite directions—you skyward, your board to Neptune's underwater world—make sure you put your hands over your head when you resurface after your spectacular dismount. This is one of the prime occasions when your board can sling-shot back at you, probably fins first. Although technically a safety maneuver to get you out of a potentially dangerous part of the wave, diving off your board is one of the most fun

∗**tip**

Beware of flying surfboards. When someone dives off a wave, their board becomes a missile, particularly if they're not wearing a leash. And if it's windy, flying boards can get blown quite a distance, often in unexpected directions. Maybe this is how "airs" were invented.

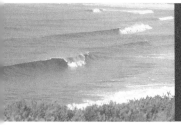

BETHANY: Remember to take the time to feel accomplished in the little things that come along the way, and not to go out with the expectation to stand up and be really good, because it won't happen and you'll end up getting injured on a beach in Mexico—which happened to me! Like today I navigated my way out of a rip; I didn't know how to do that before, and it felt really good.

things you can do in surfing. It's like a controlled wipeout. So go with it: do a frog dive or a swan dive; give a yelp or a whoop of joy!

● If the wave's small, crouch down, grab the outside edge of your board, and lean into the wave. Try to hang on to your board and let the wave break over you, making sure you stay low and really lean into the wave to stop yourself from going over with the breaking lip.

● If you're riding a shortboard or you're confident in your turns, you can turn the nose of your board into the face of the wave. This is easier on a shortboard than on a longboard because you can actually pierce the wave and get through to the other side in a kind of sideways duck dive.

Last words

Don't try too hard. You have to put in effort to learn anything new and make progress, but there's a difference between doing that and struggling to be better. If you start pushing yourself too hard, pretty soon surfing will become just another thing you have to be good at, another measure of your self-worth instead of something you really enjoy for its own sake.

Encourage yourself. You might feel like a raw beginner, but let's put your surfing into perspective. Aren't you the same person who, not so long ago, didn't know one end of a surfboard from the other? And now you're standing on a surfboard and going along beautiful green waves. While it's helpful to look ahead, it's also useful to look back now and then. The more you progress, the easier what you've learned seems to be. Which means that what you're learning now will seem easy one day, very soon . . .

Set goals. Goals don't have to be grand things. You might just want to stand up on your board for more than twenty seconds, or do a neat left-hand turn, or flick off a wave without falling off. It doesn't matter what it is, pick a move and, the next time you paddle out, practice it exclusively. The more you do it, the more it'll start to feel like second nature.

Keep learning. The great thing about surfing is that the learning never stops. As soon as you master one skill, there's another waiting in the wings, saying, "Hey, my turn!" That can seem demoralizing at first, but think of it this way: It keeps things interesting. Surfing can never get boring as long as you're paying attention.

Be yourself. Surfing's about more than trying to copy your favorite surfer. It's about bringing *yourself* to your surfing. No one else can surf like you. It's sometimes said: Leave it on the beach. Meaning: Don't take your stress and aggression out into the water with you. Sometimes, though, we leave too much on the beach with our towels. Show who you are when you surf.

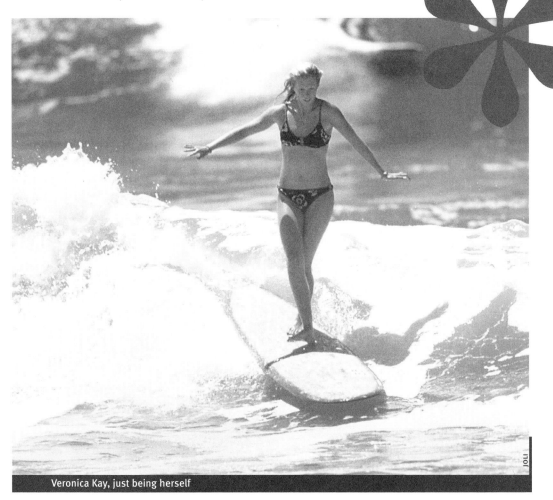

Veronica Kay, just being herself

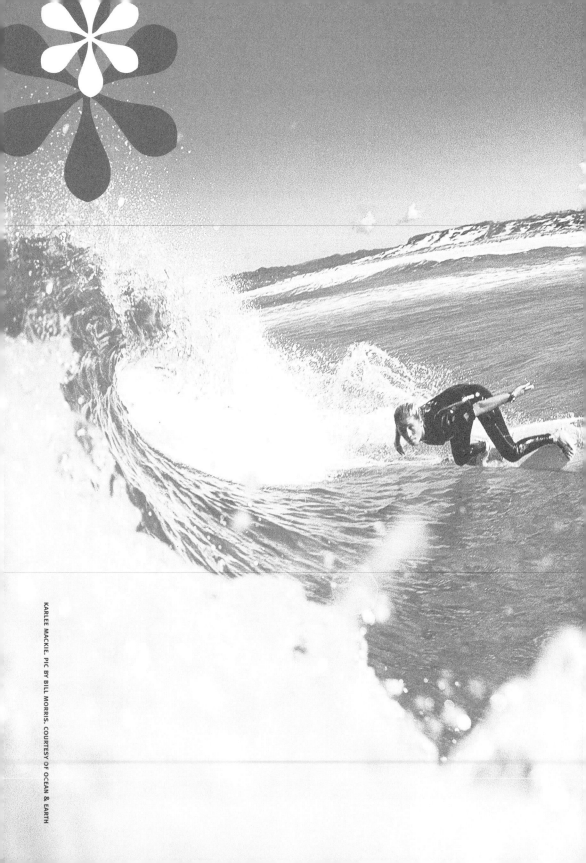

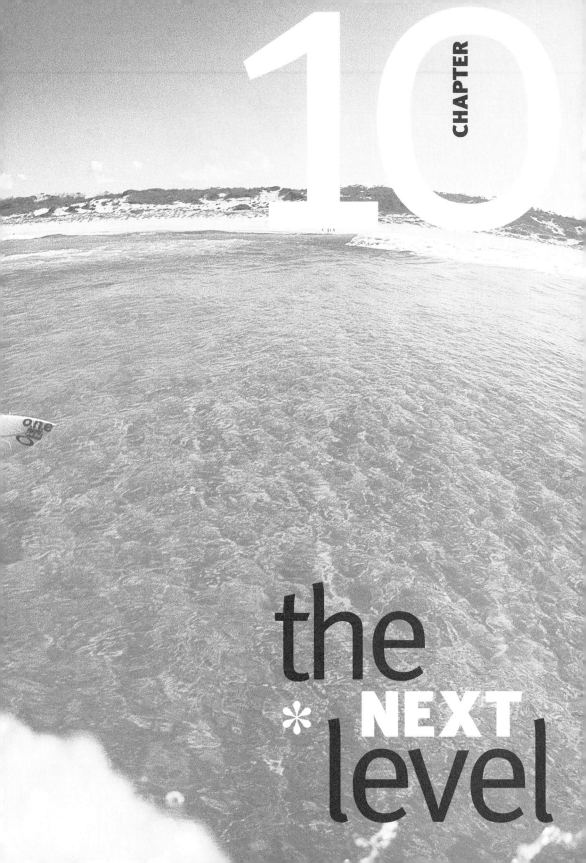

10

the
*NEXT
level

Learn:

How to tackle bigger waves. **Get into winter surfing.**
Find a surf coach. **The pros and cons of changing** your
board. How to start competitive surfing. **Where to surf**
next—the wonderful world of surf trips, including some of
North America's best surf spots.

Next stop, experience

This is an exciting time. Now that you can catch waves, stand up, and turn your surfboard, you might feel anything's possible—and it is! Or you might feel you're at a crossroads, bamboozled by all the options ahead: bigger waves, competitive surfing, surf trips. . . .

Here are a few ways to take your surfing to the next level, bearing in mind that it's perfectly okay to stay where you are for a while—by practicing what you know. Practice is the glue that sticks surfers together. Even pro surfers have to get up and go surfing on days when conditions are less than ideal and they'd rather stay in bed. Plus, you have a big advantage: Everything you practice now is new, so you can see results for the time you put in. Whichever road you choose, you're gaining more experience every time you paddle out, and that is a valuable goal in itself.

Surfing bigger waves

One of the first things you'll probably want to do when you start becoming confident in your surfing is tackle bigger waves. We're not talking Pipeline here; "bigger waves" can refer to waves that are just a little bigger than the ones you've been riding. The important thing is to know your limits—don't push yourself before you're ready—while nudging those limits aside sometimes to see if perhaps you really *can* handle those waves that you've assumed were beyond your capabilities.

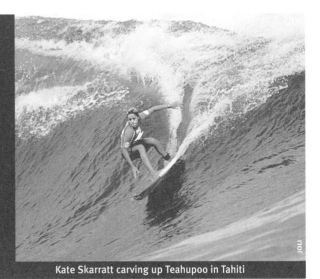

KATE SKARRATT: The first rule of thumb is knowing your ability and following your gut feeling. If you feel uncomfortable about the conditions you're about to go out in, wait a little longer or don't go out. But then the other side of it is that you often have to push yourself a little to keep progressing in bigger waves. Usually you'll have a good feeling, it's like an anticipation anxiety. If you get that, then follow your feeling and take the plunge.

Kate Skarratt carving up Teahupoo in Tahiti

Big is beautiful (and sometimes easier too)

It's a little-known fact that surfing bigger waves can be easier in some ways than surfing smaller waves. Waves that have a bigger face to ride give you more time to get to your feet before you get to the bottom. They often break in deeper water than smaller waves—so when you wipe out you've got less chance of hitting the bottom. And it's often less crowded than when the waves are small. Plus, when there's real swell, the waves come in sets—groups of waves—separated by lulls, which makes paddling out easier.

How do you know when you're ready for bigger waves?

You don't have to be a star surfer to tackle bigger waves. You just have to want to do it. One of the best ways to tell if you're ready is to think about how you're surfing now: If you're taking off on the biggest "set" waves, it shows you're ready for something a bit more challenging.

Paddling out

One of the hardest things about surfing bigger waves is getting out there. Dealing with fear on the beach and making the decision to go is one thing, but there's also the practicality of duck-diving under walls of whitewater. Get your duck-diving up to speed before you go out, and practice using your foot instead of your knee to push the tail of your board deep. Wax your rails where you hold your board so you don't lose your grip. Hold on tight when you turtle-roll; you can even wrap your legs around your board if you're afraid you're going to lose it—losing your board when the waves are solid can be scary. And if you get a chance, surf at a point break where you can paddle out through a channel instead of through the whitewater.

Tips for surfing bigger waves

- **Surf with someone more experienced than you.** You'll feel safer surfing bigger waves with someone who's more comfortable with the conditions than you are—they can show you where and when to paddle out, where to sit to avoid getting caught inside by a set, and which waves to go for. Choose your surfing buddy carefully, though; it's got to be someone you trust, who knows your surfing ability.

- **Confidence.** If tackling big waves feels like a battle, confidence is your best weapon. Fear and anxiety can do strange things to your memory; don't listen to them! Remind yourself of the times you've gone for set waves and surfed circles around your own ideas of what you thought you could do.

- **Be prepared.** As Kate Skarratt says—she took on Pipeline in Hawaii in *Blue Crush*—preparation is critical when you're tackling bigger waves: "I prepare all my equipment, make sure everything feels good—my leash, my leash string, and my wax, check there's no dings in my board. I do a bit of stretching and just check out the conditions and really make sure I know where I'm going to sit and which waves I want to take off on and not take off on. I spend a lot more time doing that when it's a bit bigger, and it puts me into a different zone—I kinda get into a bit of an excited trance. And then I talk with the people I'm going to go out with and we work out where we're going to sit and all that kind of stuff."

- **Warm up with small waves.** Give yourself a confidence boost as soon as you get out there by catching a few smaller waves. It'll warm up your muscles and get you focused as well as reminding you that, yes, you can still surf!

- **Feel the fear and go anyway.** It's normal to have fear whenever you take a step out of your comfort zone. Remember the fear you had standing up for the first time, or taking your first drop on a green wave? Facing bigger waves seems to bring out the fear in everyone—even the surfers who look so relaxed out there might still be experiencing a certain amount of anxiety. The key to coping with your fear is not denying it or trying not to feel afraid, it's just accepting it and going ahead with the game plan, like catching a wave or two. In fact, a certain amount of fear can be a positive—it makes you take the conditions seriously and pay attention. And when that adrenaline starts surging through your body, it can actually start to feel a little bit less like an anxiety attack and a little bit more like raw excitement. Go, girl!

✳ tip

Bigger waves travel faster than smaller waves, so you need to paddle harder to catch them. When you're paddling for a wave and you think you've caught it, take a couple of extra strokes just to be sure; there's nothing more demoralizing than getting caught in the lip and going "over the falls" on your first attempt at pushing the envelope.

✳

ROCHELLE BALLARD: The biggest obstacles in big-wave surfing are fear and lack of experience. Once you start gaining experience and develop your ocean awareness, your fear slowly starts to go away. Because, to me, fear is the unknown. Once you start to become familiar with something, you become less afraid of it.

LOATA'S STORY:
BIG WEDNESDAY AT COLLAROY

It was the biggest day ever, and it was a Wednesday! It was a bit of a mental challenge for me because my husband, Colin, was saying, "Maybe you shouldn't come out; it's a bit big," and I'm like, "No, I can do this!" So I start paddling, the rip is unbelievable, and eventually I get out there and I'm gasping for air, and I look across at Colin and he's yelling *"Quick!"* and doing this frantic arm-waving. Then I saw this wave surging toward me. The closer it got, the bigger it got. So I threw my board, and when I dived under, my ears were ringing so hard from the pressure. I popped up, and then two seconds later I had to go back under—by this stage I'm hanging on for dear life—and then the third wave came. I looked up and thought, I'm going to die. I had visions of the rescue helicopter pulling me out and me vomiting all over the place. So I thought I'd better grab sight of Collaroy [on Sydney's northern beaches] for the last time. And then, just as I was going to dive under the wave, I thought, No, do it properly and you won't regret it, so I went under—kick, kick, kick—and I could feel the turbulence holding me down for ages; it felt like my eardrums were going to burst, and I popped up, got on my board, and just paddled for the shore! And the whole world changed in front of me. Collaroy was just this beautiful place, and I was alive! I felt so good afterward. I got in the car and I was on a high, thinking, Wow! Near-death experience, but man, I'm going to surf well tomorrow! The next day I went out and it was only about 4 to 5 foot and I just went off—I wasn't scared, my focus was really good. I just knew, what could possibly go wrong? I was telling Colin later about the previous day, "I really thought I was going to die out there," and he said, "There's no way you would have died in that," because he'd had that experience, but I hadn't. And it didn't matter who told me, I had to experience it to know.

Beware: small surf

Although big waves (whatever that means for you) can be more terrifying than small ones, some of the worst injuries happen when you're surfing small waves.

Why are small waves so deceptively dangerous? Well, for one thing they break in shallower water. You don't concentrate as much when you're surfing in small everyday conditions as you do when you're surfing the swell of the decade. And when the waves are small, the beaches are often more crowded, which increases the likelihood of surfers and their boards hitting one another. Of course, big waves pack more of a punch and can hold you down longer. There's no answer to this paradox: just be aware that wave size is no indicator of danger.

Winter surfing

Summer may be the best time to learn to surf—the water's warm, the days are long, and if you live on the East Coast or in Southern California or Hawaii, you won't have to invest in a wetsuit—but surfing all year round is a great way to develop as a surfer. Besides, depending on where you surf, fall and winter can bring the best waves of the whole year. You don't want to miss those, do you?

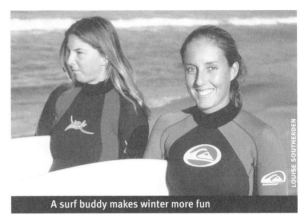

A surf buddy makes winter more fun

LOUISE SOUTHERDEN

Seven good reasons to chill out

1. **Good waves.** Sure, nothing beats surfing in warm, sparkling water, but the fact is, some of the best waves are generated by winter weather systems. Autumn is my favorite time in Sydney: the water's still warm and sparkling, the offshore winds make the skies clear and the waves perfect, and the summer crowds have gone.

2. **It's less crowded than summer.** This not only means more waves and fewer mid-ocean collisions—you don't have to worry about swimmers—it also makes you feel kinda special. Winter is a great bonding time between surfers, a time when you feel lucky to be a surfer and to be able to enjoy the water in ways that landlubbers can only dream about.

3. **Offshore winds that blow all day.** In summer, the wind is usually offshore only in the mornings and the evenings. In winter, you don't get that sea breeze phenomenon because the

BETHANY: It's hard to get motivated to go surfing when it's cold, and *it* is cold in San Francisco; you have to wear a fullsuit the whole year, even in summer. But I just try to remember that once you're in the water everything warms up and you get used to it, and I think of how I feel when I get out of the water and look forward to a cup of tea and a hot shower!

land doesn't warm up much during the day relative to night-time; plus, the weather systems that bring waves often bring offshore winds.

4. **Hot showers, hot soup, hot mugs of hot chocolate.** In fact, hot anything!—after a surf. It's not called comfort food for nothing.

5. **A sense of adventure.** There's something exhilarating about being out in the elements on a day when most people are stuck indoors beside the fire.

6. **Practice.** If you surf all year, you keep practicing your surfing and you stay fit; stopping for winter means you have to kick-start your surfing when summer comes around again, and that wastes valuable surfing time.

7. **Wetsuits.** Okay, so wearing a fullsuit makes it harder to paddle and they're a hassle to get on and off, but they do have advantages. You don't have to worry about losing your bikini top to the waves. There's no need for sunscreen anywhere other than your face (don't forget your ears!). They give you a bit of padding on your knees, hips, and ribs and protect your skin from fin chops, which can give you the confidence to try flashy moves you'd never dare in summer with all that exposed flesh. Oh, and they feel great—like an all-over body hug!

WHAT'S A CUTBACK?

A cutback is an almost 360-degree turn that takes you back to the whitewater and the power center of the wave. If you feel yourself going too far out onto the shoulder, it's time to do a cutback—that is, turn back toward the breaking part of the wave and then turn toward the direction you were traveling in before you did the cutback.

Getting a surf coach

Now that you know a few basic moves, you might want to try a few variations: cutbacks, off-the lips, re-entries (exotically called "reos"), and—let's go crazy—floaters, airs, and 360s. What you can do on your surfboard is limited only by your imagination. Oh, and a few physical laws like gravity, but hey, that never stopped anyone from trying.

There are basically two ways to take your surfing up a notch. One way is to practice what you already know, experimenting with new moves like a mad scientist, falling off, and trying them again. Before surf schools were invented, this was how everyone learned to surf—and many surfers still do it this way. But learning by trial and error has a few drawbacks: You can develop bad habits without even realizing it, and it can take a long time to progress. That's why there's another way: get a surf coach.

Surf coaching is now more popular than ever, particularly with girls. Why? "It's not that girls need coaching more [than guys], it's that girls are willing to be coached and take direction," says Mary

ALISON: I'd been surfing for about six months when I started getting coaching. I was able to stand up, I could catch the white-water, I could sort of turn. Then I did eighteen months with a surf coach, which is kind of like Finishing School for surfers, and I came out of that feeling comfortable taking off on green waves, taking off in crowds, and being able to surf in a range of waves on a range of boards.

Setterholm of Surf Academy, California's largest surf school. "For guys it's a pride thing, they want to keep things to themselves. The girls want to know what they're doing and how they can improve. They'll say to me, 'Show me how I look' or 'What's my style?' or 'How am I moving?' They're all totally into it."

How do you know when you're ready for surf coaching?

One way to tell if you're ready to get a surf coach is when you find yourself asking, "What next?" It doesn't matter what level you're at. You don't have to be into competitive surfing. Anyone and every-one can benefit from a little one-on-one attention. Basically if you want your surfing to progress and you can afford it—the going rate for a surf coach is between $50 and $80 per hour—coaching is the way to go.

What's involved?

The best thing about having your own surf coach is that you can get as much or as little instruction as you want. It can be a regular thing—two hours every weekend for a few months—or one session whenever you feel you need it. You might decide you need a few one-hour coaching sessions to work on a particular aspect of your surfing. Or you might want to use your coach as a surf buddy, to build your confidence.

So what happens in a typical surf coaching session? It all starts before you even get to the beach: Most surf coaches get the ball rolling by asking you a few questions about your surfing, your board, and any problems you might have experienced.

When it's time to hit the water, your coach will spend part of the session surfing with you, and the rest of the time on the beach, watching or videotaping you while you surf. As surf coach Mary Setterholm explains: "We don't just videotape their surfing, we videotape them paddling, sitting out in the water and trying to

BEL: I got some coaching to get someone to push me, and to correct me where I couldn't see I needed correcting. It's pushed me to get out in bigger waves. It's pushed me to put myself in situations I wouldn't normally take myself, and it helps me concentrate more on what I'm doing rather than just going out there and having a social surf.

catch waves, because often it isn't so much their surfing that needs work but the fact that they're letting good waves go by. Women especially often don't take that extra stroke to get into the wave. So we use videotaping to identify their character as a surfer and then help them develop according to their own style."

The benefits of surf coaching

Working with a professional surf coach has lots of pay-offs: improved technique, more confidence in the water, greater ocean awareness, knowing you've got the right gear to suit your surfing, and having someone experienced to surf with. It also cuts down on the time it takes to learn new moves.

According to Mary Setterholm, surf coaching helps you develop in four major areas. "There's ocean awareness: How much you know about the sea, the tides, how the wind affects the waves. Then board-handling skills: What's your stroke like? Are you holding your hand too high up out of the water? Surfing is 90 percent paddling, so if you don't have a good paddling stroke, your surfing's going to suffer. Another area is "ocean swim skills." Ocean swimming is completely different from pool swimming. If you're a good ocean swimmer, you're going to be more relaxed out in the water, you'll know how deep you need to dive when a big set comes, and you'll feel a lot safer out there if your leash breaks. The fourth and final one is surfing! So we have a lot to work on. People say "coach me in surfing" but I need to find out about these other areas and see where your strengths and opportunities are. Your surfing may really pull together if we work on your paddling stroke, because then you'll be able to catch more waves. Or if we work on your ocean swim skills, you're going to have more confidence in the water."

How to find a good coach

Some surf schools offer surf coaching as well as lessons, but before you sign on for coaching make sure your coach has worked with intermediate or advanced surfers, not just raw beginners. Word of mouth is often the best way to find a reputable surf coach. Ask your local surf shop or contact Surfing America to find out if there's a qualified surf coach in your area (see Appendix 3 for details). Then arrange a time to meet them so you can see if you both get along—it's important to find someone you can relate to, feel comfortable with, and trust—and prepare to progress!

*tip

When it's cold and rainy and the waves are no good, have a marathon chick-surf-flick afternoon with your friends. Watching girls' surf videos is a great way to get motivated, and when you're trying to learn a particular move, they give you plenty of role models! (See Appendix 3 for a list of videos.)

Changing your board

The time will come when you'll outgrow your faithful old surfboard, the board you learned to surf on, and find yourself at a well-worn fork in the road. One way leads to shorter surfboards, the other to longboards (boards over 9 foot). Why change your board? Because you'll start to feel it's holding you back. Maybe you want to do more turns or you want to try hanging five (nose-riding, not to be confused with nose-diving—you've probably done enough of that already!).

Which way to go? It's not just about which board is easier to carry (although that *is* an excellent selling point for shortboards). The fact is, both shortboards and longboards have their pros and cons. It's a matter of personal preference: What board do you feel most comfortable on and what kind of board do you feel is most suited to your style of surfing? One of the best ways to find which board suits you is to try out a few, so beg, borrow from your friends, or rent them at a local surf shop. In the meantime, consider the following pros and cons, bearing in mind that, whichever road you take, you'll probably find more pros for the board you've chosen and the cons won't matter.

LOATA: The guys in the surf shop said if you turn your body and your board doesn't go with you, it means you've outgrown your board and you need to get a shorter, thinner one. Because if your body turns and your board's going the other way, it's holding you back.

Shortboards—easier turning and duck-diving

Shortboards come in all shapes and sizes, although their distinguishing characteristics are that they're under 7 foot, with three fins and a pointy nose.

The good news: The two biggest advantages of riding a shortboard are that they turn more easily than longboards and they're easier to duck-dive, which makes paddling out less of a battle against the whitewater than what you've experienced so far, because you can slip smoothly under each wave. They're lightweight, so they're easy to carry, which is particularly good news if you have to walk or ride your bike to the beach. They fit in your car (even when it's not a station wagon), so there's no need to strap your board to the roof. It's easier to ride hollow fast waves, make steep takeoffs, and pull

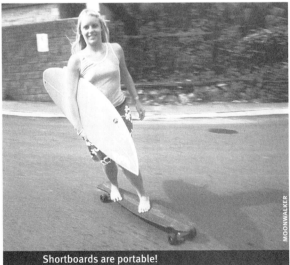

Shortboards are portable!

ESTHER: The reason I went to a shortboard was that I like to *not* feel the board: it's more just you and the wave. The advantage of a longboard, though, is that you catch more waves so you're learning more. So don't go to a shortboard too quickly. You should be catching a lot of waves before you go onto a shortboard. Surfing is about catching waves and having fun, not about the coolest board.

into tubes on shortboards, because they're shorter and less likely to nose-dive than longboards. And because they're short, they use less wax!

The not-so-good news: The things that make shortboards easier to turn also make them unstable, so you're more likely to fall off more often until you get used to balancing on one. They're harder to paddle because they sit lower in the water, instead of gliding across the surface. They're pointy (read: dangerous); put a nose guard on your board as soon as you get it. More radical surfing can mean more competitiveness among shortboarders and more impact on your knees and lower back. And finally: You can't hang ten (nose-ride) on a shortboard!

Longboards—grace and easier wave-catching

A true longboard is a surfboard that's 9 foot or longer—most are between 9'0" and 9'6"—with a rounded nose. They too come in different shapes. At the risk of oversimplifying the complex art of surfboard shaping, flatter boards are easier to paddle and nose-ride, while curvy boards (with nose and tail lift) turn more easily.

The good news: Longboards allow you to catch more waves and ride them farther—some say you can actually ride more parts of the wave on a longboard—which is their prime advantage over shortboards. They also allow you to catch waves before they get steep, so you have more time to get to your feet and get your balance before you have to make your first turn. You can surf in a greater variety of conditions—when the waves are small, big,

WHY CHOOSE?

With the recent resurgence of longboarding, the embers of the longboard-vs.-shortboard debate have been fanned into flames, with protagonists of each claiming their type of surfboard is the best. But who says you even have to make a choice? Many surfers own longboards *and* shortboards and, on any given day, they simply take out the board that best suits the conditions. In fact, there's a whole subgroup of surfers who maintain that a "real" surfer can ride any kind of board, long or short.

IZZY TIHANYI, SURF DIVA: I ride a bunch of different boards, mostly longboards like my 9'6" nose-rider with a big single fin. And right now I'm playing around with some shorter boards, especially for traveling. I'm riding a little 7'7", pretty much a shortboard for a bigger girl—I love it. And I also have a 7-foot fish [a wider shortboard] with four fins and a swallowtail; it paddles like a longboard and rides like a skateboard! It's really fun; that's better for mushy days.

smooth, mushy, slow, fast. Because they float so well and glide across the surface of the water, longboards are easier to paddle. You can even move around on the board while you're surfing, allowing you to hang ten: that is, walk up to the nose and hang your ten toes over. Surfing longboards is gentler on your body; you don't need to throw yourself around as much as you do when you ride a shortboard. Longboard surfing also has the potential to be less competitive (it feels less serious) so there can be more camaraderie between surfers.

The not-so-good news: It's more of a hassle to lug longboards around, particularly if you live in an apartment (ever tried getting a 9'6" in and out of an elevator or up and down several flights of stairs?). There's the hassle of strapping them to the roof of your car, which has two accompanying drawbacks: potential for injury (from stretchy straps prematurely released) and worry over boards being stolen when you're sitting down for a post-surf mocha and your car's parked around the corner, out of sight. They're harder to turn and less responsive than shortboards— you've got to use your whole weight. You can't duck-dive them, so paddling out in bigger waves can be a mission. If your board hits you (or someone else), it hurts more and the risk of serious injury is greater. They're also more expensive than shortboards (because there's more board!).

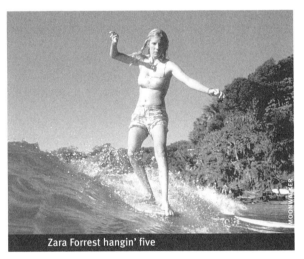
Zara Forrest hangin' five

> **BEL:** Changing my board was one of the best things I could have done. I went from a 7-foot beginner's board to an 8'6" longboard. I wanted a longboard because I live in a crowded area [Manly Beach, Sydney] and I thought, Well, at least I'll be able to catch more waves, and the more waves I get the faster I'll improve.

Competitive surfing

It's a common misconception that only "good" surfers enter surf competitions. As a result, lots of surfer girls avoid contests because they assume they're not good enough—that is, until they find out that surfing in front of other people is about more than just showing everyone how well you surf or finding out what they think of you.

So what is competing about? It's about getting to surf your local beach with only two or three other surfers in the water; how often can you do that outside of a contest? It's about improving your surfing because you push yourself harder when you're competing than when you go "free surfing" (surfing noncompetitively). Surf contests also force you to surf when conditions are less than ideal—which means you surf more than you otherwise would, and that can only help you improve. And when you're not surfing, you get to watch other girls surfing. Then there's the social side: It's fun surfing with a bunch of other girls!

"I think the biggest thing with the girls is that they don't want to get out there in front of everyone and fall off their boards and think they look like kooks," says Kathy Phillips, executive director of the Eastern Surfing Association (ESA), the largest amateur surfing association in the world. "But even [four-time world champion] Frieda Zamba started out as a kook. So just get out in the water and have fun, but at the same time, watch what other girls are doing and get as much practice time in as you can. And each time you enter a contest, if you do a little better than last time, you know you're learning."

Where do I sign up?

Competitive surfing can seem mind-boggling to the uninitiated—there are local contests and there are pro events on the World Championship Tour (WCT) that culminate in one talented woman being crowned world champion, but what happens in between? And where do you start if you want to dip your toes in the waters of competitive surfing?

Start local. A good place to start is with a local contest, like one organized by your nearest surf shop or surf school. Lots of surf contests welcome beginners, and many even have beginners' divisions.

On the East Coast, one of the best contests for first-time competitors is the annual Sisters of the Sea comp every Labor Day weekend (late August/early September) in Jacksonville, Florida. It's girls-only, there's an orientation for first-time competitors to explain how to surf a heat and how to prepare yourself, surfers

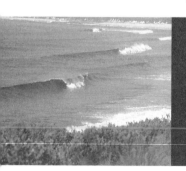

EMY: After one surf comp, you'll want to go in another one—it's so much fun and even if you do really badly, you always come out of the water laughing. You get to meet new people and whether you win your heat or you win something in the raffle, you always come away with something. It helps your surfing too because if you're a natural [regular foot] and you always surf rights, sometimes in the contests you're forced to go left, so you get better at surfing both ways.

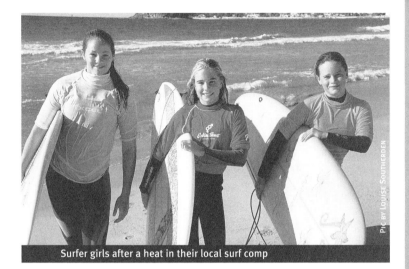

Surfer girls after a heat in their local surf comp

KARINA PETRONI: I've been a part of the ESA all my life. I started competing when I was ten or eleven. I remember at my first contest I locked myself in my room, I wouldn't go; they had to drag me out the door. Then I started winning a lot, and that gave me a lot of confidence. Then I started getting my butt kicked, but that was good too because it made me stronger. I love competing. I love that feeling of winning!

under ten can be assisted in the water (e.g., by their parents), and there's a "novice" division for "whitewater surfers" (i.e., beginners) where you're judged on how long you ride the wave.

On the West Coast, there's the League of Women Surfers (LWS), the brainchild of Mary Setterholm, former U.S. Women's World Champion and founder of Surf Academy surf school in Southern California. Each LWS event consists of surf competitions (for short-boarders, longboarders, and bodyboarders), surf lessons for beginners, and the Surf Star Clinic—video coaching for surfers of any levels designed to enhance their surf skills (participants get to keep their personalized DVD).

Go regional. If you're having fun and want to develop your competitive skills, the next step would be to join a surfing association, such as the Eastern Surfing Association or ESA (former world champs Lisa Andersen and Kelly Slater both started their competitive surfing careers through the ESA), the Hawaiian Amateur Surfing Association (HASA), the Texas Gulf Surfing Association (TGSA), the Western Region Surfing Association (WRSA), or the National Scholastic Surfing Association (NSSA). Most welcome new competitors and many have "novice" or beginner divisions—you don't have to be an aspiring pro to compete. All these organizations are now governed by the mothership of competitive surfing, Surfing America, which is a great resource for anything to do with competitive surfing. (Check out their website: www.surfingamerica.org.)

Going pro. If you can accumulate enough prize money from local comps or find a supportive sponsor to help you along, you might want to follow in the footsteps of your fave surf stars and start

WANT TO SURF LIKE A PRO?

One way to push your surfing is to go surfing with three friends, pretend you're in a big contest, and surf according to the judging criteria of the Association of Surfing Professionals (ASP):

"The surfer must perform committed radical maneuvers in the most critical sections of a wave with style, power, and speed to maximize scoring potential. Innovative and progressive surfing will be taken into account when rewarding points for committed surfing. The surfer who executes this criteria [sic] with the highest degree of difficulty and control on the better waves shall be rewarded with the highest scores."

competing in the World Qualifying Series (WQS) and, if that goes well, the World Championship Tour (WCT), where seventeen of the world's top female surfers compete for the world title. Check out the Association of Surfing Professionals (ASP) website (www.aspworldtour.com) for info on the top women pros, including ratings and contest schedules, ask pro surfers what they did to get where they are today (some of them help out at girls' surf days—see Appendix 3 for details), and, if you can manage to go along to a WQS or WCT event and watch the action firsthand, you might pick up some tips on how to make the grade.

The wonderful world of surf trips

One morning very soon, if it hasn't happened already, you'll head out for your usual surf check and decide that instead of surfing at your local beach—the beach where you learned to surf, the beach where you always surf—you're going to check the surf somewhere else, maybe even somewhere far, far away. . . .

If there's one thing that defines a surfer more than anything else, it's traveling for waves. Whether you're heading up the coast to spend the day surfing somewhere you've never been before, packing up the car for a weekend in Baja, or planning your first trip across America, to Hawaii or even farther afield, nothing beats that feeling of escape and anticipation, particularly when what lies ahead is a big unknown.

Surfing new and different spots is great for your confidence. It challenges every part of your surf repertoire, forcing you to apply your newfound skills—paddling out in the right spot and coming in safely, finding the best takeoff spot, predicting what the waves will be like tomorrow—to a totally new location. But one of the best things about surf trips is that your daily routine becomes dictated by the wind and the waves: You wake up early to surf before the onshore, or sleep in to time your surf for a higher tide. . . . It's also great fun. In fact, camping out or staying somewhere far from home with your friends, good waves at your doorstep, and plenty of time to ride them is one of the joys of the surfing life.

Where to go?

One of the hardest things about going on a surf trip is knowing where to go to find the kind of waves you want—and being able to "read" the conditions when you get there to figure out precisely where (and when) to surf. It takes practice, of course, but there are a few shortcuts you can take along the way.

- Travel with more experienced surfers who know your destination better than you do. Surfing where they surf might seem scary at first, but it can also take your surfing to a new level (particularly when your only other option when they're surfing is to sit on the beach getting bored!).
- Wander through a comprehensive surfing guide such as *The Stormrider Guide to North America* (Low Pressure). From Baja

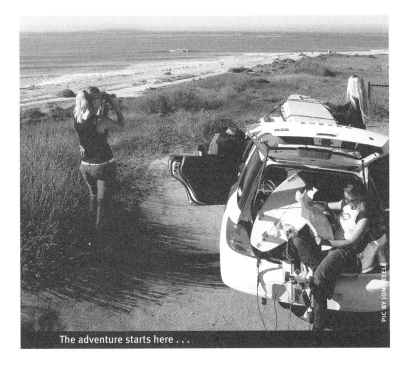

The adventure starts here . . .

LEARN-TO-SURF TRIPS

Surf trips aren't just for experienced surfers. In fact learn-to-surf trips are a great way to develop as a surfer: because you're on vacation in a beautiful setting, you're relaxed and open to new experiences, you have plenty of time to surf, the water's warm, and you're surrounded by like-minded surfer girls. Most organized trips include daily surf lessons (or instruction for nonbeginners) and yoga sessions, as well as surfing equipment, accommodations, and all meals. Some throw in a free rash guard, a massage, or private surf lessons, and optional extras can include Spanish lessons, rain forest walks, snorkeling with dolphins, whale-watching, and horseback riding along the beach. The two most popular destinations for learn-to-surf camps are Hawaii and Costa Rica:

- In Hawaii: Kelea Surf Spa combines the indulgence of a spa with the fun of surfing; Maui Surfer Girls and Swellwomen offer weeklong surf and yoga trips on Maui (for girls aged twelve to seventeen years and women aged eighteen and up, respectively); and Big Island Girl Surf Camp runs weeklong surf adventures.

- In Costa Rica: Las Olas Surf Surfaris for Women was the first (established in 1997 with the goal of turning "women into girls"!); also Del Mar All-Girls Surf Camp and Pura Vida Adventures. (See Appendix 3 for contact details.)

to Alaska, Texas to Nova Scotia, this is one inspiring guidebook. For each region there's an overview, a briefing on local surf culture, detailed maps, and a description of the best breaks. See also *Surfer's Guide to Hawaii* by Greg Ambrose (The Bess Press), and *The Surfer's Guide to Costa Rica* and *The Surfer's Guide to Baja*, both by Mike Parise (SurfPress Publishing).

- Surf the net before you go. There are loads of great websites listing surfing destinations around the world and providing up-to-the-minute surf reports for those destinations. Surfline (www.surfline.com) gives ultra-detailed descriptions of every inch of the U.S. coastline and beyond. Other good sites are www.wannasurf.com and www.surfmaps.com.

To help you on your way, here is a wandering albatross's eye view of some of the best surfing destinations within reach of most U.S. surfers, to give you a taste of the wide expanse of possibilities out there. And remember this: There are thousands more surf spots along 12,383 miles of American coastline, just waiting for you to go and find them. . . .

The East Coast

Because of its tropical climate, and because it's the first part of the coast to pick up the hurricane swells that swirl up from the Caribbean between late July and late October, **Florida** has long been considered the epicenter of East Coast surfing. The water's warm year-round, and the waves are generally friendly. The continental shelf is wider here than on the West Coast, which means that East Coast waves tend to be less powerful (waves break at the edge of the continental shelf and re-form to break on the beaches, whereas on the West Coast the swells break only once, when they get to the beach).

South Florida might have the best climate, but most swell is blocked by the Bahamas until you get to **Fort Pierce's North Jetty**, a bowling right hander on the north side of Fort Pierce Inlet. Moving north is Central Florida's most well-known and (because of that) most competitive break, **Sebastian Inlet,** a classic wave where world champs Lisa Andersen and Kelly Slater started turning heads (the nearby jetty being the bleachers). If Florida is the center of East Coast surfing, **Cocoa Beach** is the hub of Florida's surf scene; Canaveral Pier is a popular spot with local surfers.

Fort Pierce is also where the East Coast's most distinctive feature begins: the sandy barrier islands that separate the mainland from the Atlantic Ocean. Most of the best surf breaks north of there break on the outside edge of these barrier islands. In North Florida, there's **New Smyrna Beach**, on the south side of the Ponce Inlet, the most consistent wave in Florida (as Surfline.com puts it, "when the whole world is flat, you can usually find a wave here"), **St. Augustine Blowhole** (named for its hollow left-breaking barrels), and **Jacksonville Beach**.

Next on the East Coast agenda is **The Outer Banks**, North Carolina's star attraction and the holy grail for East Coast surfers. **Cape Hatteras** gets the best waves because it juts out into the Atlantic Ocean farther than anywhere else on the East Coast, making it open to any and every swell. It's beautiful and soulful, populated by craggy fishermen who have a love-hate relationship with visiting surfers. It's also one corner of the legendary Bermuda Triangle, but don't let that put you off. The waves can be glorious, especially in September when the ESA Eastern Champi-

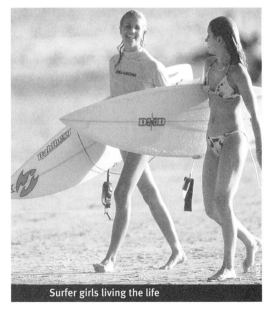

Surfer girls living the life

onships are held there. It's an adventure getting there, too—leaving the mainland and driving along the causeway, catching ferries between barrier islands that aren't linked by road, and ending up at Buxton's stripey lighthouse feeling like it's just you, the ocean, the birds, and those fishermen. . . .

Continuing north, the Intercoastal Highway is the surfer's Yellow Brick Road leading you to the next well-known surf spot: **Manasquan Inlet, New Jersey**, at the mouth of the Manasquan River (athough there are waves all along the Jersey shore, and it's not as polluted as people assume). Between Labor Day and Memorial Day you can basically surf anywhere, anytime, but come summer (with its swarms of tourists), New Jersey makes life difficult for surfers with "beach badges" required at many spots (you have to pay for access to the beach and wear a badge on your swimsuit or boardshorts), metered parking, even fees to use restrooms and showers, and at some beaches surfing is banned altogether during daylight hours.

Might as well keep traveling north . . . to **Long Island, New York**. There's more than one hundred miles of surfable, south-facing coastline between Coney Island in Breezy Point, Brooklyn, and Long Island's most easterly extremity, Montauk. Some of the best waves can be found along the jetties of Rockaway Beach and Long Beach, and the pristine sands of Jones Beach, Gilgo Beach, and Fire Island. Montauk is one of the few areas on the East Coast with a rock bottom, which gives reeflike precision to many of the breaks such as Ditch Plains (great for longboarders), Atlantic Terrace, and Turtles. Because these breaks are the most exposed to swells from all directions, surfers will often talk about how big the surf is in Montauk, as an indicator of how much swell is reaching the rest of Long Island (the waves are always bigger "out east," i.e., between West Hampton and Montauk).

If you're really serious about your surfing, you won't let a little thing like the cold stop you getting into **New England**'s waves (just bring plenty of rubber: booties for most of the year, and you'll need gloves from October and hoods from late fall to late spring). It's a beautiful part of the world with twisting coast-hugging roads, heart-stopping cliffs, and dramatic changes of season that color the forests. Best of all, geological features such as slabs of granite, cobblestones, and boulders on the sea floor give the waves shape and allow the breaks to handle solid swells. **Narragansett Beach, Rhode Island,** is a popular spot. **Ruggles** is another, but don't let its cuddly name fool you: It's known mainly for being able to hold sizeable swells. **Cape Cod**'s beach breaks are fickle but can turn it on, especially on the National Seashore near Eastham. Farther north, if you can find waves in New Hampshire and Maine (the swell's mostly blocked by Nova Scotia in the north and Cape Cod to the south), you'll probably have to share them with only a few locals and a seal or two. Over the border, **Nova Scotia** has a wonderfully convoluted coastline that forces southerly swells to wrap around points and into sheltered bays and a big wave spot to call its own (the Bay of Fundy).

When to go (East Coast): Hurricane season, late July to late October, when big swells that originate in the Caribbean swirl up the coast giving surfers a reprieve from summer flat spells. In winter, low-pressure systems offshore can bring idyllic surfing conditions, but be prepared for the cold water anywhere north of Maryland. The East Coast gets big seasonal variations in water temperature compared to the West, especially in New England: by late summer you can surf in a bikini and boardshorts as far north as Maine, but in winter it's fullsuits, hoods, booties, gloves, and snowdrifts on the beach!

The West Coast

When surfers say "the West Coast," it's actually code for "California." Sure, the Pacific Northwest, BC, and Alaska can get perfectly good waves at certain times, but the cold and the general wildness of the ocean most days make them off-limits for all but the most hardy surfers.

California, on the other hand, is a road trip waiting to happen. The Pacific Coast Highway leads you scenically through every beach town, providing surf-check opportunities while you drive in some places. It also has a few classic ingredients that make its waves the envy of other coastlines. Hot, dry Santa Ana winds blow offshore in summer and fall, smoothing the surface of the ocean

OVERSEAS SURFARIS

Picture yourself in a far-off land. It's warm all day and balmy all night, there's never more than five other surfers in the water, and the only decision you have to make each day is whether to surf twice or three times. Sounds cool, huh? Ready to hear about all the places where you can make this dream surf trip a reality? Well, there's Puerto Rico, Mexico, Costa Rica, Hawaii, Chile, Brazil, Barbados, the Maldives, the Philippines, Bali, the Mentawais, Java, Lombok, Sumatra, New Zealand, New Guinea, Fiji, Tahiti, Tonga, Samoa, Sri Lanka, South Africa, France, Portugal, Spain, Ireland. . . . Wherever land meets sea, virtually, there's the possibility of waves. It's a big wide surf-blessed world out there. For a glimpse of all the overseas options, check out www.wannasurf.com—it lists more than 3,500 surf breaks in eighty-four countries (including the U.S.), as well as surf reports, swell and wind forecasts, and surfing news.

and making for great surfing conditions. Even when the wind does go onshore, kelp beds keep the waves smooth and glassy. The coastline is varied enough that when it's onshore and flat on one part of the coast, it's probably offshore and pumping not too far away. There's always that promise of the perfect wave, if only you can find it.

There are literally thousands of named surf breaks between **San Diego** and **Santa Barbara,** where Southern California unofficially ends and Central California begins. Some of the most consistent spots are in San Diego County, particularly around **Sunset Cliffs,** where there are a dozen or so reef breaks set against steep cliffs—the only way to get to the beach is to carry your board down the steep path that surfers have beaten over the years. Some, like New Break, a beautiful right-hander, involve climbing up and down a rope. **Tormaline,** sandwiched between Pacific Beach and La Jolla, is a lovely beginner-friendly wave.

Heading north past the beach towns of Ocean Beach, Mission Beach, and Pacific Beach, **La Jolla** is home to Windansea and Big Rock—the Sunset Beach and Pipeline of the West Coast, heavy in terms of both waves and locals. Then there's **Black's**, a clothes-optional beach since time began, and one of the best beach breaks in America; not only that but the time and effort required to negotiate the cliffs to get to the beach keeps the crowds down. **Seaside Reef** offers a consistent right and left, then **Cardiff Reef**, a long right-hand longboard wave that breaks gently over a grass-covered reef, making it ideal for families wanting to surf together. Half a mile north, **Swamis** (so-named because of the nearby Self-Realization Center in Encinitas) and **Leucadia** mark the end of the southern reef breaks and the beginning of the beach breaks like Carlsbad and Oceanside.

Orange County surfing begins with **San Onofre,** a good spot for beginners and a gathering place for SoCal longboarders. Less than a mile up the beach, you'll come to another famous break: Upper and Lower **Trestles**. Trestles has always had a love-hate relationship with surfers. Most surfers are attracted by its consistency, although others feel the reason it's consistently mentioned in surfing magazines is that it just happens to be on the doorstep of America's most prestigious surfing publications: *Surfer, Surfing*, and *SG*.

Continuing through Orange County, you come to the famous **Huntington Beach**, where big city meets beach town and creates something of a "surf city." Huntington is home to the U.S. Surfing Championships, great beach breaks, and the famous Huntington Beach Pier, where you can slalom between the pilings. Most visitors surf near HB Pier, while locals tend to surf Huntington Cliffs and other less-hyped spots.

Although it gets super-crowded, every surfer must, once in her lifetime, make a pilgrimage to **Malibu**, the legendary right-hand point break where Gidget learned to surf. It's simply one of the best small-wave breaks in the world. If the crowds get too much, just enjoy the spectacle of every man and his dog (literally!) surfing the perfect peeling waves. Otherwise, head to nearby **Zuma Beach** or the more beginner-friendly **Topanga Beach**. Halfway between Ventura and Santa Barbara there's another famous right-hand point break: **Rincon,** where rides of 300 yards are not uncommon.

Although Northern California doesn't technically begin until you're halfway across San Francisco's Golden Gate Bridge, most surfers (especially the ones that live and surf there) will tell you that **Monterey Bay, Santa Cruz**, and **Half Moon Bay** (home of big-wave surf spot Mavericks) are NorCal. Maybe it's an identity thing—there is something hard-core and soulful about surfing in Northern California. Or maybe they just want everyone to know how cold the water is: There's a reason O'Neill wetsuits were born in Santa Cruz. Whatever the reason, be prepared for attitude to match the water temps at **Steamer Lane**, the main surfing spot in Santa Cruz. Incidentally, there's a surf spot underneath the Golden Gate called **Fort Point**, and it's best during big winter swells when the waves at San Francisco's more exposed ocean beaches like, er, **Ocean Beach**, are too big and messy.

When to go (West Coast): Unlike the East Coast, which relies primarily on seasonal hurricanes for wave action, the West Coast gets its swell primarily from prevailing westerly winds any time of year—with the wind strength, and wave size, increasing the farther north you go. In winter the most solid ground swells come from the north.

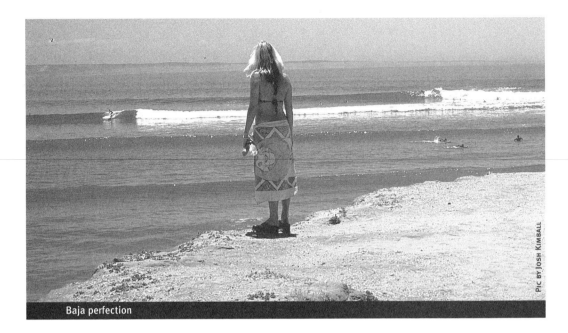

Baja perfection

PIC BY JOSH KIMBALL

Baja California, Mexico

There's no sweeter sound than the words "Let's go to Baja" issuing forth from your best friend's lips. It's California without all the people, it's the desert mixed in with a little Latino culture, it's tacos and practicing your Spanish, and it's perfect waves. If you live in Southern California, "Lower California" is close enough for an impromptu surf trip: downtown Tijuana, Baja's largest city, is just ten minutes from downtown San Diego. You can even do a day trip from L.A. to Ensenada, Baja's second-largest city.

For a short trip, stay north of **Ensenada**. Northern Baja has dozens of beach and reef breaks and right-hand point breaks to quench your thirst for waves, like K38s, "K38 and a halfs," and K55s (so named because that's how far they are, in kilometers, from the border). Then there's San Miguel and Las Gaviotas. Isla Todos Santos (Killers), the famed big-wave spot, is down there, too, accessible by boat from Ensenada.

If you've got more time, and a reliable vehicle, hit the Trans-Peninsula Highway (Mex Highway 1) and discover some of Baja's more closely guarded secret spots. The end of the road is almost 1,000 miles from the border, at **Cabo San Lucas** (known to visiting surfers as simply Cabo), a little fishing village at the southernmost tip of Baja. If funds aren't in short supply, you can fly there. The living is easy in Cabo, with long days spent surfing Monuments (near town) or The Rock (a popular longboarding wave), exploring nearby artists' villages, and sipping margueritas as the sun goes down over the sea, ending with long nights dancing and partying (if you're not exhausted from those long days).

When to go (Baja): Anytime. Summer can get crowded, especially in Northern Baja, and the water can be surprisingly cold, thanks to strange currents that bubble up from underwater canyons. The best waves come in fall. A word of warning: If you rent a car in the U.S., you might not be able to take it into Mexico, and don't go to Baja without travel insurance.

The Gulf Coast

Although it does get waves in hurricane season, the Gulf Coast—including the west coast of Florida and the coastlines of Alabama, Louisiana, and Texas—is not somewhere you'd go for a surf trip unless you live nearby. But if you and your surfboard do find yourselves there, **Texas** gets the best waves of the Gulf, because it's on a more direct path for the hurricane swells coming up from the Caribbean via Yucatan. The surf spots of choice are around Corpus Christi, Padre Island, and Galveston Pier (which is popular with surfers from Houston). Less consistent but still very surfable waves can be found at Mussel Shoals, **Alabama**, before heading along the Florida side of the Gulf of Mexico (where pro-surfing brothers Cory and Shea Lopez hail from), although most Florida surfers move to the East Coast for more consistent waves.

When to go (Gulf Coast): Hurricane season, late July to late October. The water's almost tepid in summer, and beware of the natural oil deposits that bubble up in the summer months—they can coat the deck of your board (not to mention you) in a sticky goo.

Hawaii

Hawaii's North Shore, on the island of Oahu, 2,000 miles from mainland USA in the middle of the Pacific Ocean, has been a mecca for surfers since time (and surfing) began. It's a place where legends are made and boards (and spirits) broken, where "localism" was virtually invented, and where many surfers still go for their baptism of fire in terms of challenging waves. Prime big-wave time is winter, but there's more to Hawaii than huge waves and heavy locals. In fact, Oahu can be a pretty fun place to surf, especially in the summertime.

And there's more to the North Shore than **Pipeline, Backdoor, Sunset Beach,** and **Waimea Bay**. In fact, on this strip of coast barely six miles long, there are more than twenty-five different spots to surf. **Monster Mush** and **Kammiland** can attract the same size swells as the more well-known spots, and because they

> **ROCHELLE BALLARD:** Everybody thinks of Hawaii as a winter surfing destination, but the summertime's fun, too, particularly on the south shore of all the islands. There's not as much power in the waves, but it's still beautiful water.

break gently over reefs, they can give visiting surfers a taste of big-wave riding. **Pupukea** and **Beach Park** are popular spots for North Shore surfer girls (Hawaii has lots of girls who rip), and from there it's only a twenty-minute walk up the beach to get a glimpse of the action at Sunset, the famous right-hander and one of Layne Beachley's favorite waves. Pipeline is another good wave-watching spot because it breaks so close to the beach.

Beyond the North Shore, Oahu's west side is longboard heaven and Honolulu is learn-to-surf city (although Diamond Head has some worthy reef breaks). In particular, Publics and Queens, both off **Waikiki Beach,** get perfect waves that seem to carry you ever-so-gently to shore—just be prepared to share your ride with a variety of other craft, from catamarans to outrigger canoes. Beyond Oahu, there are plenty of options, too (be prepared to pay extra to take your surfboards on some interisland flights): **Kauai, Maui,** and **the Big Island (Hawaii)** all have surf spots galore set amid one of the most lush and awe-inspiring landscapes you will ever see: rain forest–cloaked mountains, spectacular waterfalls, volcanoes, black-sand beaches, and an ocean filled to the brim with marine life. Hawaii occupies a special place in the hearts of anyone who has ever surfed there, and there are two keys to enjoying your experience there: respect the locals at all times, and soak up that Aloha spirit.

HOME SWEET HOME

I feel at home when I'm sitting on my green board with my feet dangling in the water, looking at the horizon, watching for the shadow that hints of a wave. The sea birds have better things to do—gannets that spear into the water from a fearsome height and bob back to the surface with small silvery fish in their beaks, and seagulls riding the wind that follows the contours of each wave, up and over, inches close to the water. But I'm just waiting, with the other surfers. We sit in silence, each in our own thoughts. I wonder if they notice the way the sun catches the drops of water on their eyelashes and gives them stars in their eyes. Or how green the water is today. Or the sound of water running over the deck of their surfboards. Or the feel of tiny jellyfish against their fingers when they paddle. Do they like the way the waves smooth their hair when they duck-dive, how it feels to be caressed by the sea from head to toe? Maybe they do. Maybe they wonder if I do. Each of us is in the same world but feeling in our own worlds, like circles that intersect where we speak about the waves and the direction of the wind as it starts to come onshore and the tide that's now so low that sand explosions accompany every breaking wave. And when I catch my last wave in and drop down to my belly to ride the whitewater before stepping off into shallow water, releasing the Velcro strap around my ankle, and walking up the beach to the shower, I'll look back to where I was, out there, and feel the privilege of being a surfer.

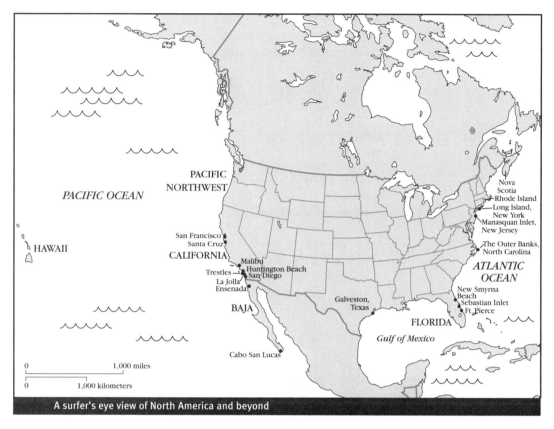

A surfer's eye view of North America and beyond

The road from here

If the journey of a thousand miles begins with one step, technically it also ends with one; at least it does when your destination is a fixed place. In surfing, however, there is no destination—or, rather, it keeps shifting. This can feel pretty frustrating when you're starting out, but the truth is, it's what makes surfing such a lifestyle. And if you keep surfing and putting your time in, before long you'll realize something else: You haven't just learned to surf, you've become a surfer.

What does it mean to be a surfer? To me, it's waking up in the morning and sticking your head out the window to check which way the wind's blowing before you even go to the bathroom. It's finding sand in the oddest places: under the couch cushions or in the pockets of your jeans. It's driving the long way round, past the beach, even when you're in a hurry with no prospect of ocean time that day, just because you have to know what the waves are doing.

It's getting to work with wet hair and your boss looking sideways at you because he knows why you're late. It's sitting in your old station wagon at your favorite beach on a rainy Saturday afternoon, peering past the sweep of your windshield wipers just to make sure you're not missing anything. It's living in a house where it doesn't matter if your feet are sandy. It's choosing a bikini not just for how good it looks, but for how well it stays on in the surf. It's standing on the headland with your arms folded and your hair going crazy in the wind, watching a too-big swell throw itself against the rocks. It's surfing with your loved one and loving the way the water droplets cling to his eyelashes. Or leaving town at a moment's notice—throwing your board and your tent in the car, picking up your best friend on the way, and heading up or down the coast in search of good uncrowded waves.

Being a surfer is feeling like you're in on this great secret and knowing that wherever you go in the world, if you meet another surfer, you'll always have something to talk about. Last but not least, it's feeling respected by other surfers, and respecting them in return, because we all know what it takes to be a surfer.

Whatever surfing and being a surfer means to you, it's yours to enjoy. So put your time in, go surfing whenever you can, and embrace the surfing lifestyle, and may it give you some of the best days of your life.

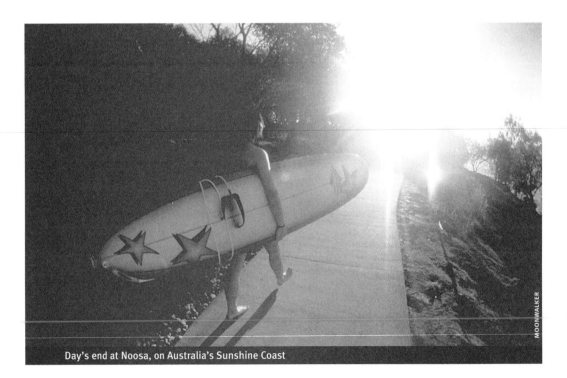

Day's end at Noosa, on Australia's Sunshine Coast

the
surfer*
girls

Angie Gosch

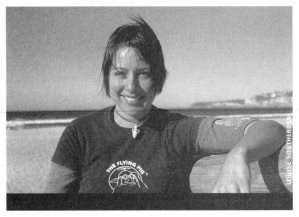

Angie grew up six hours' drive south-west of Sydney, Australia, in the Snowy Mountains of New South Wales, but learned to swim at the age of two—her parents used to call her "the fish." So when she moved to Sydney a few years ago, she gravitated to the beach and started surfing "because Manly Beach and the northern beaches have become so much my home, and surfing is such a large part of the culture, and the sea just calls to you all the time to come and play!" She rides a 6'2" Jim Banks single fin.

"I began surfing because my ex-boyfriend was a surfer and he was really into it, surfed every day. So I used to go out with him but that was hopeless, because he was so addicted he didn't have enough time to really teach me. Then, after he and I broke up, I borrowed one of his boards, which was the Jim Banks; it was something I had to do myself. Now I've got such a passion for it. I love just being out there in the elements. It's an adrenaline rush, knowing that you can never truly be in control because it's nature and it can change at any moment."

Belinda (Bel) Glynn

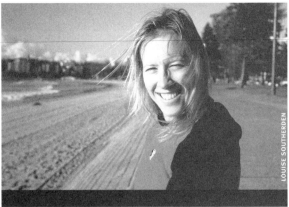

Bel is a regular in the surf at North Steyne on Sydney's Manly Beach—she just walks down to the beach from her apartment in Manly, with her 8'6" O'Donnell under her arm. She's been surfing for two years, and recently opted for night shift at the law firm where she works so she could live the surfing life during the day.

"I think there's an untouchable factor about surfing: that you completely lose yourself in it, and it can be totally unreal. It has added a completely different dimension to my life. I can't think what I used to do on Saturday and Sunday mornings before. Did I really just go to the supermarket and shop? I did yoga and stuff, but there was nothing that gave me the thrill and the adrenaline rush. It completely highlights your life, gives it color and depth. You see little animals out there, like fairy penguins or fish or stingrays; it's just unbelievable."

Esther Hamburger

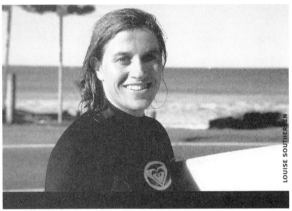

Esther moved to Sydney from the Netherlands four years ago in pursuit of a guy: Rogier (also Dutch and now her husband). She didn't know much about the ocean back then but was keen to learn, so she started body-boarding. Within a month, she'd trans-ferred to a 7'8" mini-longboard and taken a few surf lessons. She now rides a 7-foot Feisty and a 9-foot McTavish Firebird. She and Rogier live in an apartment with a panoramic view over Curl Curl Beach on Sydney's northern beaches, so checking the surf in the morning is as easy as sitting up in bed!

"Surfing makes me feel so good! And you're really in that little world. . . . For me it feels really good to be so concentrated on one thing, and all the stuff that's happening outside of that is gone. . . . Also, I'm clumsy on land, but in the water I'm not. I think it's from being more mindful in the water. And when you're surfing, you're really busy with your balance, and it's all about the changing envi-ronment and reacting to it. I like to be aware of my body, and surfing really, for me, keeps my mind and my body in the same place."

Emy Tesoriero

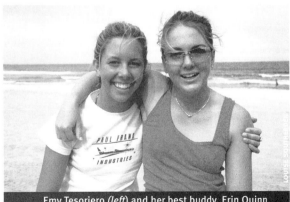

When Emy was nine, she joined her local surf lifesaving club at Dee Why Beach, Sydney, and met another girl who loved the water as much as she did. They became best friends and started surfing about two years ago, when they were both thirteen.

Emy lives at Bilgola Beach, Sydney, and surfs after school at Dee Why or Warriewood. She had about ten surfing lessons when she started, and now rides a 5'10" Luke Short.

Emy Tesoriero *(left)* and her best buddy, Erin Quinn

"The thing I love about surfing is being able to do it and people envying you because it's something not many girls do, and the boys look up to you if you're out there and not just sitting on the beach. You get a rush from it. You can be free in the water. I think of it as a kind of meditation, a kind of relaxation time, when the adrenaline's not pumping from it being so big!

Alison Aprhys

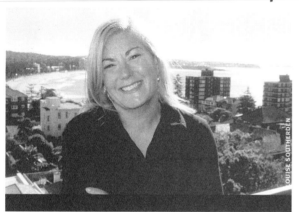

Before Alison discovered surfing on the windswept beaches of Victoria, on Australia's chilly south coast, she was a dedicated career woman: a communications consultant and freelance journalist who "lived in high heels, all black, and red lipstick." Then she started surfing, and her wardrobe, not to mention her lifestyle, changed. She now lives in an apartment overlooking Manly Beach with her husband, Peter, her vast collection of shoes (which now includes several pairs of stylish flip-flops) and her four surfboards: a pink and orange 7'2" Corey Graham, a 7'4" McTavish Carver, which she calls her "little black dress of surfing—if I don't know what to ride I'll take that out"; a Fish (a wide shortboard for surfing small waves); and a 9'1" McTavish.

"I started surfing when I was thirty-eight. It changed my life, because I was looking for an activity that would really, really make me happy. I fenced for ten years competitively and I was good at it, but rheumatoid arthritis in my knees got the better of me. Then one day at the beach I said to Peter, a longtime surfer, 'Why are we at the beach? It's raining and it's July [winter in Australia],' and he promptly enrolled me in a surfing class and I was hooked. So I quit working full-time and took up freelancing so I could surf more often. One of the reasons I came to Sydney was that a company offered me a contract up here and I told them I'd come as long as I could live near the beach!"

Loata Sanderson

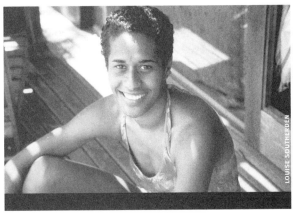

Loata grew up in Suva, Fiji, and went to Australia when she was seventeen. She and her family lived in western Sydney, far from the beach, where she went to university. Finally, after she graduated with a Bachelor of Nursing, she returned to the sea by moving to Manly Beach, to work for the Department of Community Services helping people with intellectual disabilities, often working afternoon shifts in order to surf in the mornings. She learned to surf on a 6'2" McCoy (a thick shortboard), now rides a 6'8" Pipedream, and lives at Newport with her husband, Colin (also a surfer), and seven-year-old daughter Savannah, who has already had a go at surfing on her mom's board!

"When I first had this vision that I was going to be a surfer, I imagined myself riding down to the beach on my bike with a board under my arm; that was my dream. It was all about the image. But being a surfer takes away the vanity. Now I'm concentrating so much on what I'm doing, I even forget about having matching stuff! My whole life has changed. It doesn't matter if it rains, hails or shines; as long as the waves are good, I'm happy. I listen to the weather reports more than I've ever done before, on the radio or TV. And what I do in my spare time has changed: I'm not interested in going shopping at all now. All I'm interested in is going for a surf or being around the water or watching people surf. Obsessed, I think the word is!"

Bethany Currin

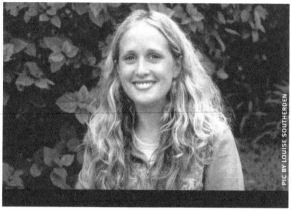

PIC BY LOUISE SOUTHERDEN

The first time Bethany got on a surfboard, she had probably the worst wipeout of her surfing life. She was on holiday with her family in Todos Santos, a little Mexican town at the southernmost tip of the Baja Peninsula, and decided it was time to learn to surf. "It was my birthday, and all I wanted to do was go surfing. I had so much confidence; I'd seen a million surf videos. I didn't think I needed a lesson or anybody to show me anything; I just rented a board and paddled out. But obviously, never having had a surf lesson, I didn't know what to do when a wave came, so my board came up and hit me in the face and my tooth went through my lip. I went underwater and tasted blood right away. And the next day I had to have five stitches in my lip, which was scary in a Mexican hospital!"

A year and a half later, after her wounds and her confidence had healed, she was back out there, this time under the watchful gaze of her new boyfriend Wes, whom she met in her hometown, San Francisco. Unfortunately it was January, but she couldn't wait any longer, so she rented a board and a wetsuit—"but no booties, it was freezing!"—and they surfed Half Moon Bay, just south of the city. Now Bethany rides a 7'6" board that Wes shaped for her, surfs as often as she can, and whenever the cold water threatens her motivation, she just reminds herself how she feels after surfing. "I'm always so exhilarated after a surf. Usually tired and hungry, but I feel so good and my body feels alive. It's a good feeling."

Deborah Stoll

Although Deborah grew up in Florida, her first surfing experience came when she was living in Manhattan; she and her snowboarding girlfriends decided to have a surf lesson at Montauk, Long Island. "It was one of those things—like snowboarding and traveling—that I'd spent so much of my life having this kind of unconscious perpetual longing. I just woke up one day and realized I was sick of reading about it; I wanted to do it!" Two years later, after Deborah made the big move to sunny California (she writes TV shows and film scripts

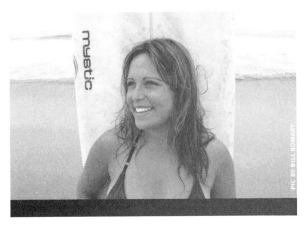

for a living), her older brother presented her with her first surfboard for her birthday, a custom 9-foot Mystic longboard; and she now lives five minutes from "surf central," Malibu Beach.

"My life has completely changed since I started surfing. I walk around in flip-flops and cutoff jean shorts, I carry my board, my wax, and my wetsuit in my car all the time! My schedule is totally different. All my friends kinda laugh at me because I'm a city girl but now I stay home and try to go to bed by eleven or twelve so I can wake up early and surf. I just really love it. One of my favorite things with surfing is when you walk out into the water, and the first time you lie down on your board, almost the second your feet leave the sand, you're in a completely new space. It's really beautiful."

Anna Cooper

Surfing began as a way for Anna to make new friends when she moved to Jacksonville, Florida, from Tallahassee (two and a half hours from the coast) three years ago to finish her degree in psychology. And although she is something of an ocean girl—she learned to bodyboard at the embryonic age of four when her family was living in Hawaii, and she's a keen scuba diver, a qualified lifeguard, a swimming and aquarobics instructor, and she coaches a swim team in Jacksonville—she had

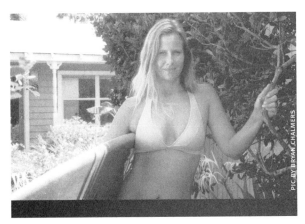

never tried surfing before. "I'd always wanted to do it, but when I was growing up it just wasn't something that girls did. I would sit on the beach and watch the boys that I was dating surf." Now she rides a 7'6" funboard, surfs almost every day across the road from her house at Jacksonville Beach with her girlfriends, and, helps out at Sisters of the Sea and ESA surfing contests up and down the East Coast.

"Learning to surf is probably the best thing that has ever happened to me. I love the feeling of total freedom and the independence of surfing. I love the ocean, its power and unpredictability. It brings you peace, because you have to just let go; you can't control it. You have to be totally in the moment, and that's what I love about it. I've made great friendships with people of the same mind-set. And I feel great after every surf, regardless of what happened; whether I got tumbled, or I turned, or got stuck in a rip, I still feel great. I feel so alive."

Kaitlyn Margeson

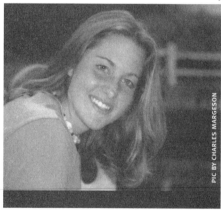

PIC BY CHARLES MARGESON

When Kaitlyn goes surfing, she doesn't have to worry about fitting her surfboard in the car or looking for a parking space at the beach or hiding her car keys while she's out in the water—because her nearest surf beach is a fifteen-minute boat ride from her house in Amityville on New York's Long Island. All she has to do is throw her 7'3" Bic surfboard into her twenty-foot open boat, cast off from her backyard jetty, and motor across Long Island Bay to Fire Island. Although she got her first taste of surfing when she was little, Kaitlyn didn't really get into it until she was fifteen years old when she took up bodyboarding. A year later, she made the transition to a surfboard but still keeps her bodyboard "for when the surf's really big." Then she joined a surfing club run by her high school chemistry teacher who, Kaitlyn says, has been surfing "forever." They watch surfing movies through winter and go surfing after school and on weekends in summer at Gilgo Beach, Long Island.

"What I really love about surfing is that it helps you to know not just the ocean but the whole ocean environment. And I love how surfers are all part of this great big community. I'm so happy to be in that community now, to know a whole bunch of surfers, and to get into the whole outlook on the environment. I am so much more comfortable in the ocean now. I could surf for the rest of my life."

surf
lingo

Like any subculture, surfing has its own language, and understanding and learning to use it is part of learning to surf. Of course, language is always evolving—you and your friends might even make up a few new words yourselves—so the following is an introduction to surfing terminology, divided into sections to make it easier to find words.

How's the surf?

One of the easiest ways to check the surf is to ask someone when you get to the beach. The hard part comes when they answer. That's when it helps to know what they mean when they say its . . .

blown out   The waves are messed up and made generally unrideable by strong onshore winds.

clean   Ideal surfing conditions, making it easy to distinguish one wave from the next.

closing out   The waves are collapsing all the way along their length instead of peeling; that is, they are closeouts.

double overhead   Each wave is about twice as high as the surfer riding the wave.

epic   Basically the best surfing conditions imaginable, usually used when the waves are at least overhead; also, firing, pumping.

fast   The waves are breaking like a fast-moving zipper.

flat   No surf.

full   There's a lot of water in each wave, making them appear "fat" and therefore not steep enough to catch unless you're surfing on a longboard; often coincides with high tide.

glassy   The ocean and the waves are as smooth as glass, because there's no wind.

head high   Each wave is about as high as the surfer riding it.

hollow, sucky   The waves seem to fold over on themselves, often forming a hollow tube.

inconsistent   The waves are breaking unpredictably and not coming in regular sets.

maxing out   The swell is too big and the waves unrideable.

mushy   The waves are crumbling and lack power, making them uninviting to all but the most wave-hungry surfers.

✳tip
Surfers can tell a fake a mile off, so don't use a word if you don't know what it means. And don't call anyone "dude"!

offshore The wind is blowing from the land (literally *off the shore*), which smoothes the waves and makes them easier to ride.

onshore The wind is blowing from the sea (literally *onto the shore*), which makes the sea chaotic and the waves messy-looking and more difficult to ride.

overhead The face of each wave is higher than the average surfer's height. Sometimes used more specifically as in "2-foot overhead" or "a little overhead."

perfect Similar to "epic" but without the size factor; perfect waves can be any size. Sometimes, however, the conditions can be perfect (no wind and the right tide), but the waves aren't cooperating (there's no swell).

three foot Depending on the wave-measuring system you use (see Chapter 4), this means the waves are either about waist high (if you measure the face of the wave) or head high.

Other wave-related words

No two waves are the same but, like butterflies, there are lots of ways to classify them:

A-frame A wave that can be ridden by two surfers simultaneously, one surfing to the right and one surfing to the left.

backing off When the tide is so high the waves can't break.

backwash Waves that move from the beach (instead of toward the beach) and back out to sea, making the incoming waves wobbly and difficult to ride; often happens at high tide.

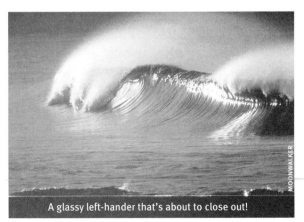

A glassy left-hander that's about to close out!

beach break A surf spot where the waves break over sand.

bomb A wave that's bigger than all the others coming through.

break, surf break A surf spot.

cleanup set A group of big waves that washes all the surfers in the water toward the beach.

closeout A wave that breaks simultaneously along its entire length, preventing you from riding it (unless you're happy just to practice your take-

offs!) because there's nowhere to go when you stand up. Sometimes a wave will peel from one end to the other at first, and then
close out, or dump.

dumping   Waves that are breaking heavily and suddenly.

ground swell   Well-formed waves generated by strong winds
that have blown over a great distance, allowing the waves to pick
up energy and get organized into neat lines before they reach your
local surf spot.

heavy, gnarly, hairy   Used to describe anything dangerous or
intimidating; e.g., "a heavy paddle" refers to a difficult paddle out,
"heavy locals" are surfers who dominate a particular surf break.
"Gnarly" can also mean "really bad," as in "That was a gnarly
wipeout, girl."

left, left-hander   A wave that breaks to the left from the surfer's
point of view (it breaks to the right if you're looking from the
beach).

lines, corduroy lines   When the crests of approaching waves
form horizontal stripes on the ocean; usually an indicator of a new
ground swell.

low, low pressure   A weather system often associated with
changeable weather that can generate waves. (High pressure
systems, or "highs," are usually associated with fine, stable weather
and are often not wave-generating.)

peeling   A wave breaking evenly from left to right, or vice versa,
like a zipper closing.

point break, point   A surf spot where the waves break around
a point.

reef break, reef   A surf spot where the waves break over a bed
of rocks or coral; usually more powerful and predictable than a
beach break.

right, right-hander   A wave that breaks to the right, from the
surfer's point of view (it breaks to the left if you're looking from
the beach).

sandbars   The mounds of sand on the sea floor that determine
bottom contours and therefore wave shape.

swell   Storm-generated bumps in the ocean before they form
waves that break.

Victory at Sea   Big, wild surf usually caused by a confusion of
wind, currents, and swells coming from every conceivable direction.

wind swell   Waves produced by local winds; these waves are usually closer together, more disorganized, and weaker than ground swells.

The anatomy of a wave

barrel, tube   The hollow part inside some breaking waves. (Getting barreled is the ultimate experience in surfing.)

bottom   The ocean floor; also the lowest part of the wave and the underside of a surfboard.

channel   Deep water where no waves break, and therefore a good place to paddle out or stay safe (not a good place to catch waves, though).

curl   The breaking part of a wave, most often heard in 1960s beach movies when people talk about "shooting the curl," or riding the wave just ahead of the barrel.

current   Moving water. The two most common are sideshore or longshore currents, which move parallel to the beach (literally *along the shore*), and rips, which move out to sea. Undertows are another kind of current, most commonly affecting swimmers; unlike rips, which move across the surface, undertows move underwater and can pull you under and out.

crest   The highest point of a wave, opposite to the trough (the lowest point).

face   The part of the wave that you ride, and the part you can see from the beach, as opposed to the back of the wave, which is only visible to surfers sitting on their boards behind the breaking waves.

green room   Another word for the barrel.

impact zone   Where the waves are breaking, usually detectable by whitewater (not a good place to linger).

inside   Used to describe where you are relative to the peak ("She was on the inside of me" means she was closer to the peak than I was) or to the beach (an "inside reef" is closer to the beach than an "outside reef").

lineup   The place where surfers sit on their boards, forming something of a line, to wait for waves.

lip   The leading edge of a breaking wave and the part of the wave that can hurt you the most if it breaks on you. On the other hand, if the lip breaks *over* you (and the wave is hollow enough) you can get tubed. Also refers to the place you put gloss and zinc (your lips!).

lull   A pause between sets when no waves break.

outside, out the back   Calm water on the ocean side of the impact zone, where surfers wait for waves. Also used to describe where you are relative to the peak ("She was on the outside") or the beach (an "outside reef").

"Outside!" or "Out the back!"   If someone calls this out in the surf, it means there's a wave coming that's bigger than the previous ones, it's going to break farther out than where everyone is sitting, and you should probably start paddling for the horizon!

paddle   To propel your surfboard forward by lying down on it and moving your hands through the water one after the other.

peak   The place you catch waves, where waves literally form a peak or bump in the water.

period   (Not what you think!) The elapsed time between two consecutive waves, used by surfers to predict swells. Wind swell— waves generated by local winds—generally has a shorter period (usually less than ten seconds) than ground swell (waves generated by distant winds).

pocket   The most desirable place to be on a wave because it's closest to where the wave is breaking and therefore has the most power.

rip or riptide   A mass of water traveling out to sea, used by surfers when paddling out.

set   A group of waves, separated by a pause, or lull.

shorebreak   Waves that break/dump right onto the beach, often dangerous to surf because they break in very shallow water.

shoulder   The gentle ramplike part of the wave that is about as far from the breaking part of the wave as you can get while still actually riding it.

Surfers and other creatures

brah   Slang for "brother" (not something you wear for support). Derived from *bruddah*, a Hawaiian word for brother.

bodysurfer   A surfer who surfs without a surfboard, the original form of surfing.

chick   A once-derogatory term now embraced by girl surfers.

dolphin   Our mentor when it comes to flowing with the waves.

Gidget   The nickname of California's original surfer girl, Kathy Kohner, who brought surfing to the attention of mainstream America in the late 1950s via *Gidget* books, movies, and TV shows.

goofyfoot   A surfer who surfs with her right foot forward.

grom, gremmie, grommet   A kid who surfs better than you (basically, a cheeky young surfer). Derived from "gremlin" (a mischievous gnome).

hard core   A surfer who is dedicated to the surfing lifestyle almost to the exclusion of everything else.

kook   Derogatory word for a beginning surfer of any age; also someone who has an exaggerated opinion of his or her own surfing ability.

local   A surfer who lives at a particular surf break, surfs there regularly, or has surfed there longer than you (an ambiguous term).

regular foot   A surfer who surfs with her left foot forward; also called *natural*.

sea urchin   A little ball of trouble that inhabits the crevices of rock platforms and reefs; its sharp spines can inflict a surprising amount of pain when stepped on. One good reason why surfers often wear booties to walk over rocks or reefs.

shaper   Someone who makes surfboards.

switchstance, switchfoot   Someone who can surf with either foot forward, the surfing equivalent of being ambidextrous although much harder, and therefore very cool. Also used to describe the act of surfing the opposite way from how you usually surf—if you're usually a goofyfoot and you ride a wave with your left foot forward, you're surfing switchfoot.

wahine   Hawaiian word for "female surfer."

Maneuvers

backside   Surfing with your back to the wave. Also called "backhand."

bail, bail out   Slide off your board when you're paddling out to dive under an oncoming wave instead of duck-diving or turning turtle. Also refers to the act of jumping off your board midride when you realize the wave is about to close out.

bottom turn   The first turn you do, at the bottom of a wave.

burn   To drop in on someone. As in, "That guy burned you bad."

caught inside   When you get caught inshore of wave after wave of whitewater, either because you're paddling out and didn't make it out the back in time or because a set came and you were sitting too far in, too close to the beach.

cutback   A turn, usually performed when the wave you're riding slows down, that takes you back toward the more critical, breaking part of the wave.

dawn patrol   Surfing at sunrise when the waves are glassy and relatively uncrowded.

drop   The vertical ride down the face of a wave; "nice drop" is a compliment on how well you handled the takeoff.

drop in   Catching a wave that another surfer has already caught—that is, stealing another surfer's wave. Also refers to dropping down the face of a wave, particularly a big wave.

duck dive   A technique that allows you to get through the whitewater by pushing your surfboard under the oncoming waves.

eat it   Wipe out.

fade   Surf toward the breaking part of a wave, the intention being to reach a more critical and therefore more challenging part.

floater   A maneuver that involves surfing over the breaking part of the wave, like a grind in skateboarding.

frontside   Surfing facing the wave. Also called "forehand."

get out   Paddle out beyond where the waves are breaking, as in "How did you get out so fast?" Also used to mean getting out of the water, returning to the beach.

go in   Enter or get out of the water, depending on the context. If you say, "Are you going in?" and you're on the beach, it means "Are you going in the water?"; if you say the same thing when you're already in the water, it means "Are you going back to the beach?"

going off   Surfing radically, as in "You were going off out there today." Also used to refer to the surf, as in "It's going off."

go out   Enter the water, go into the ocean. "Are you going out?" means "Are you going surfing?"

hang five   Walk to the nose of your surfboard and hang the toes of one foot over the edge.

hang ten   Walk to the nose of your surfboard and hang the toes of both feet over the edge; also called "nose riding."

hog, wave hog   Someone who catches more than their fair share of waves.

hold down   When you're held underwater, usually after a heavy wipeout.

hoot   An exclamation of encouragement often used when watching another surfer riding a good wave.

kick out   End your ride by turning your board through or over the back of the wave.

late takeoff   Catching a wave at the last possible moment, when the wave is at its steepest and just about to break.

over the falls   An embarrassing maneuver that involves being caught in the lip of a wave as it breaks, so you literally go "over the falls" with it.

pearl, nosedive   When the nose of your board buries itself in the water (so called because you and your board go deep underwater, as if you're pearl diving).

pop-up   The act of standing up on a moving surfboard; also called *jump-up*.

pull in   Tuck into the tube. You can also pull in to closeouts, but you won't come out the other end as you would in a real tube.

re-entry   A radical top turn that results in your surfboard pointing vertically down the wave as if you're doing a second takeoff.

rip   Surf radically; also called *shred, carve*.

snake   Paddle inside another surfer (closer to the peak of a breaking wave than the other surfer), effectively giving you right of way on the wave. Common in crowded lineups, this is the antithesis of respect and wave-sharing. Also refers to a surfer who regularly snakes.

snap   Break a surfboard, as in "I snapped my board"; also refers to a quick turn.

stoked   Excited about surfing—or anything!

straighten out   Ride a wave straight to the beach; usually performed when a wave shuts down, leaving you nowhere to go, or when you're coming in to the beach at the end of your surf.

take off   The moment you stop paddling and stand up on your board to drop into a wave; also used as a noun, as in "nice take-off."

tombstoning   When you wipe out, usually in big surf, and your board surfaces before you do—your leash pulls the tail of the board down (to where you are, at the other end, still underwater) and the top half of your board sticks up in the air like a tombstone.

top turn   The turn you do at the top (high part) of a wave.

tow-in surfing   When surfers use Jet Skis to tow them into waves that are too big to paddle into. One surfer rides behind the Jet Ski standing up (like waterskiing), then lets go of the tow rope when on the wave.

trim   Adjust your position on the wave or on your board in order to maximize speed and stay in the "sweet spot" of the wave.

tubed   The state of grace when you're inside the belly of a wave. Also: slotted, pitted, barreled.

turtle roll or turning turtle   A technique for getting through the whitewater by flipping your board upside down and hanging on underneath until the wave has passed.

washing machine   Whitewater, particularly when there's a lot of water moving around; "going through the rinse cycle" refers to a bad wipeout.

wave sharing   When surfers take turns catching waves out of respect for one another and a willingness to keep the lineup friendly.

wipe out   Fall off your surfboard. Also used to describe the act of falling off, as in "That was a spectacular wipeout!"

worked   Tossed around during a wipeout. Also pummeled, hammered, axed.

yo! yeah!   Something you can call out to another surfer when you think they're going to drop in on you (or if they already have dropped in on you) to let them know it's your wave.

Surf gear

boardshorts   Shorts made specifically for surfing. Also called *baggies* and *surf trunks*.

bodyboard, boogieboard   A foam-core belly board. Bodyboard is the generic term; boogieboard is a spinoff from the Morey Boogie, the original brand invented by Tom Morey in 1971. Also called *sponge, shark biscuit, tea bag*.

buoy   A float in the ocean that's fitted with sensitive meteorological instruments that measure wind, weather, and wave data; surfers often access this data online to determine the size and direction of approaching swells.

deck   The top of your surfboard, the side you lie on.

ding   An injury to your surfboard, usually where the fiberglass has been damaged.

fin   Used to control the direction of your surfboard; also refers to bodyboarders' flippers.

fin chop   A cut caused by a surfboard fin.

fin system   Detachable surfboard fins such as Fin Control System (FCS) that allows you to remove fins for easy traveling and change them to experiment with different sizes.

foam   What surfboards are made of (underneath the hard fiberglass coating); also refers to whitewater.

fullsuit   A wetsuit with long arms and long legs, worn all year round in Northern California, but elsewhere mostly in winter.

funboard, funshape   A surfboard that's longer than a shortboard and shorter than a classic longboard, giving it advantages of each: easier to paddle than a shortboard, but easier to turn than a longboard.

gun   A surfboard designed for riding big waves, usually longer than a regular shortboard, and with a narrow tail.

hood   A wetsuit cap that covers the head, neck, and ears, worn for warmth when surfing in cold water.

kneeboard   A surfboard that is meant to be ridden kneeling down. Usually shorter and wider than conventional shortboards.

leash, surf leash   A polyurethane umbilical cord that connects you to your surfboard by a Velcro strap around the ankle of your back foot.

longboard   A surfboard over 9 foot. A mini-longboard, usually between 7 and 9 foot, is the ideal beginners' board.

nose guard   A silicon tip that you glue onto the nose of your surfboard to keep it from poking into your eye or someone else's when you wipe out.

quiver   A surfer's collection of surfboards for different conditions.

rail   The side edge of a surfboard, the part that digs into the water when you turn.

rash guard, rash vest   A Lycra top that surfers wear for sun protection and to guard against rashes caused by lying on a surfboard or wearing a wetsuit.

shortboard   A surfboard under seven feet long, usually with a pointy nose.

softboard, soft-top surfboard   A surfboard made out of polyethylene like a bodyboard; the kind of surfboard used by most surf schools.

spring suit, shortie   A between-seasons wetsuit with short arms and short legs.

stringer   The strip of wood that runs down the center of a surfboard to give it strength.

tail   The back end of a surfboard.

tail pad, deck grip   A piece of nonslip rubber that you stick onto the tail of your surfboard instead of using wax, for extra grip when you're surfing.

thruster   A surfboard with three fins of equal size.

wax, surf wax   The stuff you rub onto the deck of your surfboard to stop you from slipping off when you lie, sit, or stand on it. Available in blocks or bars, it's not generally required on softboards.

wax comb   A piece of plastic with a serrated edge on one side and a bladelike edge on the other, used for roughing up and removing wax from a surfboard.

A bit of Aussie lingo

banks   Short for *sandbanks*, the Australian word for sandbars, mounds of sand on the ocean floor that determines wave shape.

bluey, bluebottle   A floating blue jellyfish with stinging tentacles that can get tangled in your leash and give you nightmares about duck-diving and coming up with them all over your face! A familiar sight on Australia's east coast, particularly in summer.

boardies   Boardshorts. Derives from the common Australian practice of shortening words and ending them with an "ie" sound, as in wettie (wetsuit), sunnies (sunglasses), rashee (rash guard), leggie (short for legrope, the Aussie word for leash), and shorey (shore break).

bombora, bombie   An offshore reef that usually only breaks when there's a big swell.

cozzie, togs, swimmers   Bathing suit.

the early   The dawn patrol (surfing at sunrise), as in "Let's get up for the early tomorrow."

Malibu   A longboard, or surfboard more than nine feet long. Derived from California's Malibu Beach, the birthplace of modern surfing.

mini-mal   Short for mini-Malibu (a short Malibu surfboard), it's usually about seven to eight feet long. Most beginners in Australia learn to surf on mini-mals.

Noah   Shark. Derived from rhyming slang: Noah's Ark=shark.

shack   A tube or barrel, as in "Did you see Libby get shacked on that last wave?" Also called a *keg*.

steamer   A wetsuit with long arms and long legs, usually worn in winter; also called a fullsuit.

straight hander   A closeout.

thongs   Flip-flops.

wettie warmer   The practice of peeing in your wetsuit to keep warm in winter.

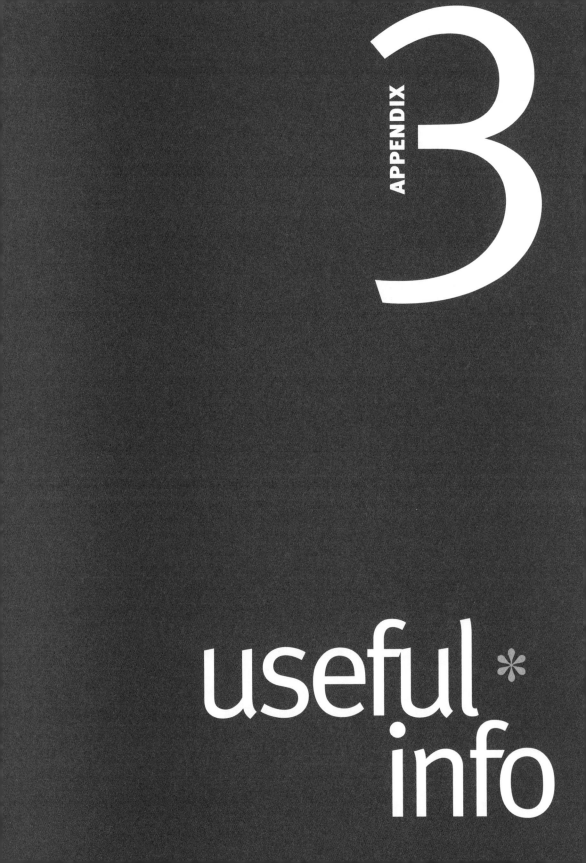

APPENDIX

3

useful *
info

Those are more resources for surfer girls now than ever before: all-girl surf schools and surf camps, learn-to-surf days, women's surf shops and magazines, websites, movies, and surfing associations. The best way to find out what's happening in your area is to get down to the beach and talk to your fellow surfer girls. In the meantime, here are a few contacts to get you started. . . .

Surf schools

Surf Diva Surf School
2160 Avenida de la Playa
La Jolla, CA 92037
Ph: (858) 454-8273
Fx: (858) 454-8505
E-mail: askadiva@surfdiva.com
www.surfdiva.com

HB Wahine
18854 Coolwater Lane
Huntington Beach, CA 92648
Ph: (714) 596-2696
Fx: (310) 244-2744
E-mail: hbwahine@msn.com
www.hbwahine.com

Saltwater Cowgirls Surf Camp
408 13th Avenue South
Jacksonville, FL 32250
Ph: (904) 242-9380
www.saltwatercowgirls.com

Surf Sister Surf School
1180 Pacific Rim Hwy.
Tofino, BC
Canada V0R 2Z0
Ph: (250) 725-4456
Toll free: 1-877-724-SURF (7873)
E-mail: info@surfsister.com
www.surfsister.com

girlsAdventureOUT
1750 Francisco Blvd., Suite 5
Pacifica, CA 94044

Ph: (650) 557-0641
E-mail: surfing@girlsadventureout.com
www.girlsadventureout.com

Swell Times Surf School

(Run by Mary Hartman, who set up Girl in the Curl surf shop in 1997)
34116 Pacific Coast Hwy., Suite A
Dana Point, CA 92629
Ph: (949) 661-4475
www.girlinthecurl.com

Surf Academy

(Run by Mary Setterholm, 1972 U.S. Women's Surfing Champion)
811 N. Catalina Avenue, #2316
Redondo Beach, CA 90277
Ph: (877) 599-SURF (7873)
Fx: (310) 372-1036
E-mail: mary@surfacademy.org
www.surfacademy.org

Pacific Surf School

721 Ormond Court
San Diego, CA 92109
Ph: (619) 742-2267
E-mail: emiliano@pacificsurf.org
www.pacificsurf.org/camp/surfgirl.html

Surf City Surf School

(Owned and operated by Kim "Dangerwoman" Hamrock, eleven-times U.S. national champion)
P.O. Box 3013
Huntington Beach, CA 92605
Ph: (714) 898-2088
E-mail: dangerwoman@earthlink.net
www.dangerwoman.com

Florida Surf Lessons

145 Morning Dew Circle
Jupiter, FL 33458
Ph: (561) 712-8871
E-mail: info@FloridaSurfLessons.com
www.floridasurflessons.com

Sunset Suzy
P.O. Box 825
Haleiwa HI 96712
Ph: (808) 781-2692
E-mail: sunsetsuzy@hotmail.com
www.sunsetsuzy.com

Nancy Emerson School of Surfing
358 Papa Place, Suite F
Kahului
Maui, HI 96732
Ph: (808) 244-7873 or 662-4445
Fx: (808) 877-4922
E-mail: nancy@surfclinics.com
www.surfclinics.com

All-girl learn-to-surf days and camps

Op Girls Learn to Ride Clinics
Girls-only action sports clinics that tour the U.S. and Canada teaching girls of all ages the basics of surfing as well as snowboarding, skateboarding, motocross, wakeboarding, BMX, and mountain biking. For schedule of events and registration, go to the website www.opgirlslearntoride.com or call (949) 499-GLTR (4587).

Rochelle Ballard's Surf Camp for Chicks Who Rip
A three-day surf camp for girls aged eight to ninteen held in Hawaii and hosted by pro-surfer Rochelle Ballard. It's free, but participants are asked to donate $45 to Boarding for Breast Cancer and International Women's Surfing (IWS). Rochelle also hosts one-day surf camps at Huntington Beach, California, and Cocoa Beach, Florida. For more info, go to www.sgmag.com, www.oneill.com, or www.rochelleballard.com.

Serena Brooke Day
An annual surf day hosted by pro-surfer Serena Brooke at Huntington Beach, California, and Jacksonville Beach, Florida. Surf lessons and contests for all ages. For more info: Sisters of the Sea (ph: (904) 247-3495 or www.sistersofthesea.org) or www.sgmag.com.

Prosurfcamp

Learn to surf or improve your skills by surfing with four-time world champion Lisa Andersen at Cape Hatteras, North Carolina. Three-day all-inclusive surf camps for girls aged ten and up. Contact: Board Sports Management at (321) 777-9935 or go to www.prosurfcamp.com.

Billabong Summer Sessions Surf Camps Tour

Billabong team riders such as Keala Kennelly, Belen Connelly, and Sanoe Lake tour the East and West Coasts and, along with surf schools at popular beach locations, offer instruction and tips. Go to www.billabonggirls.com.

Roxy Surf Camps

One-day surf camps held every summer (July–September) for girls aged seven–eighteen years, all along the West Coast, starting in San Diego and ending in Santa Cruz. Cost includes surf lesson, lunch, and Roxy goodie bag. Go to www.roxy.com.

The Betty Series Here We Go Again Tour

The Betty Team—comprised of eight surf, snow, and skate girls—visit more than sixty locations along the East and West Coasts on the Betty Bus, demonstrating surfing, skating, snowboarding, and other adventure sports and hosting surf clinics for girls. Go to www.thebettyseries.com.

Annual Wild Woman Waterday

Held over one weekend every August, this women's surf day run by Surf Academy at Surfrider Beach in Malibu, California, combines surfing lessons and surfing contests, paddleboard races, and ocean swims. Go to www.surfacademy.org.

Cannon Beach Surf All Girls Surf Clinic

A three-day clinic including surf lessons with Kim "Dangerwoman" Hamrock at Cannon Beach, Oregon. For more info, call (503) 436-0475 or go to www.cannonbeachsurf.com.

Surf trips for women

Kelea Surf Spa

Named after a Hawaiian chiefess who gave up her royal status to live by the ocean and go surfing, Kelea Surf Spa offers five-day vacations in Hawaii (February–April) and Costa Rica (Novem-

ber–January), including surf lessons, yoga classes, and spa treatments.
Ph: (949) 492-SAND (7263)
E-mail: info@keleasurfspa.com
www.keleasurfspa.com

Maui Surfer Girls

Ten-day surf camps on the west shore of Maui, Hawaii, for teenage girls aged twelve–seventeen. Other offerings: mother-and-daughter surf camps, the weeklong Surf & Yoga Experience, surf lessons, and four-hour surf clinics available Mondays–Fridays.
P.O. Box 1158, Puunene
Maui, HI 96784
Ph: (808) 280-8165
Toll free: 1-866-MSG-2002
E-mail: info@mauisurfergirls.com
www.MauiSurferGirls.com

Swellwomen

Sister company of Maui Surfer Girls, offering a seven-day Surf & Yoga Experience for women 18 years and up. Includes surf lessons, yoga, and other healthy pursuits such as massages, rain forest walks, and snorkeling.
P.O. Box 1294
Puunene, HI 96784
Ph: (808) 579-8211
Toll free: (800) 399-MAUI (6284)
E-mail: info@swellwomen.com
www.swellwomen.com

Big Island Girl Surf Camp

Weeklong surf adventures for girls and women of all ages on the Big Island of Hawaii. Activities (apart from surfing and surf lessons) include snorkeling with dolphins, whale-watching, and outrigger-canoe sailing.
P.O. Box 10452
Hilo, HI 96721
Ph: (808) 326-0269
E-mail: admin@bigislandgirlsurf.com
www.bigislandgirlsurf.com

Las Olas Surf Safaris for Women

Weeklong surf trips in Costa Rica between November and June. Cost includes accommodation and meals, daily surf lessons, use

of all surf equipment, free rash guard and sports bottle, daily yoga sessions, massage, and a private one-on-one surf lesson.
991 Tyler Street, #101
Benicia, CA 94510
Ph: (707) 746-6435
Fx: (707) 745-2261
E-mail: info@surflasolas.com
www.surflasolas.com

Del Mar All Girls Surf Camp
All-girl surf camps from three days to three weeks in Playa Hermosa, Costa Rica, incorporating surfing, yoga, hiking, and massage.
Ph: (506) 385-8535
Fx: (506) 487-8265
E-mail: info@CostaRicaSurfingChicas.com
www.costaricasurfingchicas.com

Pura Vida Adventures
Seven-day surfing adventures for women in Malpais on the Pacific Coast of Costa Rica. Cost includes beachfront accommodation and meals, daily surf lessons (instruction for experienced surfers), yoga sessions, day trips to secret surf spots, and a one-hour massage.
9186 Sebastiani Way
Sacramento, CA 95829
Ph: (415) 465-2162
E-mail: info@puravidaadventures.com
www.puravidaadventures.com

Women's surf shops

HB Wahine All Girls Boarding House
301 Main Street, #102
Huntington Beach, CA 92648
Ph: (714) 969-9369
www.hbwahine.com

Surf Diva Surf Shop
2160 Avenida de la Playa
La Jolla, CA 92037
Ph: (858) 454-8273
Fx: (858) 454-8505
E-mail: askadiva@surfdiva.com
www.surfdiva.com

Girl in the Curl Surf Shop
34116 Pacific Coast Hwy., Suite A
Dana Point, CA 92629
Ph: (949) 661-4475
www.girlinthecurl.com

Paradise Surf Shop
3961 Portola Drive
Santa Cruz, CA 95062
Ph: (831) 462-3880
Fx: (831) 462-3431
www.paradisesurf.com

Water Girl Surf Shop
23 E. Main Street
Los Gatos, CA 95030
Ph: (408) 399-5105
E-mail: watergirl_surfshop1@hotmail.com

Real Surf Shop
1101 South Coast Hwy.
Oceanside, CA 92054
Ph: (760) 754-0670
www.realsurfshop.com

Trixie Surf
Handmade surfboards for girls (and girls at heart) of all levels,
designed and shaped by Shawn Ambrose. You can custom order
fabric and artwork for your new board and even watch your new
board taking shape in the Real Surf Shop at Oceanside, California.
www.trixiesurfboards.com

Rock'er Board Shop
12204 Venice Blvd.
Mar Vista, CA 90066
Ph: (310) 397-8300
Fx: (310) 397-8931
E-mail: rockershop@earthlink.net
www.rockerboardshop.com

Girl Next Door Surf Shop
1020 Anastasia Blvd.
Saint Augustine, FL 32080
Ph: (904) 461-1441
www.surf-station.com/gnd

Surfer Girl & Guys Too
7209 Coastal Hwy.
Ocean City, MD 21842
Ph: (410) 723-6767

Rawskin Surf N' Sport
796 Carlsbad Blvd.
Carlsbad, CA 92008
Ph: (760) 434-1122
www.rawskinsurf.com

Women's surfing groups/associations

International Women's Surfing
Established by pro surfers Rochelle Ballard, Layne Beachley, Kate Skarratt, Megan Abubo, and Prue Jeffries in 2000 to further the development of women's surfing at all levels. New members welcome.
26811 Eastvale Road
Palos Verdes, CA 90274
E-mail: womenssurfing@hotmail.com
www.womenssurfing.org

Boarding for Breast Cancer (B4BC)
Nonprofit, youth-focused foundation whose mission is to increase awareness about breast cancer, the importance of early detection, and the value of a healthy lifestyle, and to raise funds for breast cancer research.
6230 Wilshire Blvd., #179
Los Angeles, CA 90048
Ph: (323) 571-2197
E-mail: email@b4bc.org
www.b4bc.org

The Betty Series
The largest sports organization for women in the courtry, offering a series of events all over America, from learn-to-surf clinics to the Betty Series of contests for all levels.
P.O. Box 510815
Melbourne Beach, FL 32951
Ph/Fx: (321) 455-2297
E-mail: bettyseries@cs.com
www.thebettyseries.com

Sisters of the Sea
A nonprofit women's-surfing association based in Jacksonville, Florida, and formed in 1997 to provide a way for women to surf together. They organize social surfings days and contests for girls and women.
www.sistersofthesea.org

East Coast Wahines
Organizers of the East Coast Wahine Championships, a two-day surfing event for girls featuring pro/am longboard, shortboard, bodyboard, and novice contests, and surf clinics, held every August in Wrightsville Beach, North Carolina.
www.eastcoastwahines.com

Ocean Divas Surf Club
An informal women's-surfing group based in Manasquan, New Jersey. Contact Joanne Dannecker or Joanie Sapienza at (732) 528-3365.

Nor Cal Women's Surf Club
San Francisco–based club that organizes a range of events, from social surf days and surf trips to surf-contest-skills clinics and more formal events like the annual Norcal Women's Surf Fest in Pacifica, California.
www.ncwsc.com

Women's International Longboarding Organization (WILO)
P.O. Box 867
Cardiff by the Sea, CA 92007
E-mail: juliecox19@hotmail.com
www.wilsurfing.com

Women's surfing contests

- **The Betty Series.** Call (321) 455-2297 or go to www.the bettyseries.com
- **East Coast Wahine Championships.** Go to www.eastcoast wahines.com
- **Girls Only Surfing Classic.** Annual amateur contest held at Fort Pierce, Florida, in October. Contact Cheryl Williams at (772) 562-5964.
- **Norcal Women's Surf Fest** in Pacifica, California. Hosted by the Norcal Women's Surf Club. Go to www.ncwsc.com
- **Wahine Surf Series.** A series of women's contests through-

out California run by Western Region Surf Association (ph (949) 369-6677, www.wrsa.org)

● For more events, go to www.bettybelts.com (Betty Belts is a Santa Cruz–based surf apparel company that sponsors women's surfing events.)

Competitive surfing organizations

League of Women Surfers
811 N. Catalina Avenue, Suite 2316
Redondo Beach, CA 90277
Ph: (310) 372-2790
Fx: (310) 372-1036
E: mary@womensurfers.org
www.womensurfers.org

Surfing America
8672 Florida Street, Suite 201-B
(P.O. Box 309)
Huntington Beach, CA 92648
Ph: (714) 848-8851
Fx: (741) 848-8861
www.surfingamerica.org

Eastern Surfing Association (ESA)
P.O. Box 582
Ocean City, MD 21843
Ph: (866) SURF-ESA or (410) 213-0515
Fx: (410) 213-2397
E-mail: info@surfesa.org
www.surfesa.org

National Scholastic Surfing Association (NSSA)
National office (see website for Hawaii, Florida, and New Jersey offices):
P.O. Box 495
Huntington Beach, CA 92648
Ph: (714) 536-0445
Fx: (714) 960-4380
E-mail: jaragon@nssa.org
www.nssa.org

Hawaiian Amateur Surfing Association (HASA)
PMB 822, 150 Hamakua Drive
Kailua, HI 96734
Ph: (808) 262-2488
www.hasasurf.org

Texas Gulf Surfing Association (TGSA)
Ph: (713) 975-5314 (North Division: north of Victoria, Texas)
Ph: (361) 937-WIND (South Division: south of Victoria)
www.tgsa.org

United States Surfing Federation (USSF)
(The organization that runs the annual U.S. Surfing
Championships in California)
E-mail: croatan@infionline.net
www.surfusa.org

Western Region Surfing Association (WRSA)
(Organizes the Wahine Surf Series)
P.O. Box 6033
San Clemente, CA 92674-6033
Ph: (949) 369-6677
Fx: (949) 469-0405
E-mail: director@ussfwesternregion.org
www.ussfwesternregion.org

International Surfing Association (ISA)
5580 La Jolla Blvd., PMB 145
La Jolla, CA 92037
Ph: (858) 551-5292
Fx: (858) 551-5290
www.isasurf.org

Girls' surfing videos and DVDs

- *Surfer Girl* (1994). The first women's surfing movie, a 16-mm documentary made by former pro surfer Debbie Beacham and Donna Olson, and featuring former world champions Frieda Zamba, Wendy Botha, and Pam Burridge, as well as Beacham and Jodie Cooper surfing perfect waves in Tavarua, Fiji.
- *Blue Crush* (1998, Billygoat Productions, www.billygoat distribution.com). Before *Blue Crush*, there was . . . *Blue Crush*!

This is the original surf film (Universal Studios bought the name from producer Bill Ballard for the 2002 Hollywood movie). Includes surfing in Samoa and Africa and interviews with pro surfers.

- *Peaches* (2000, Billygoat Productions). A sequel to *Blue Crush* (the Billygoat Productions one) that features Keala Kennelly at Teahupoo in Tahiti, Layne Beachley tow-in surfing Hawaii's outer reefs, and Rochelle Ballard's fearless tube-riding in Indonesia. Shot all over the world, in waves of all shapes and sizes, and featuring more than fifteen surfer girls.
- *Our Turn* (2000, XX Productions, www.xxproductions.com). Girls' snow, skate, and surf movie created by Californian snowboarders Sky Rondonet and Tiffany Sabol to celebrate women in action boardsports.
- *7 Girls* (2001, XX Productions). Seven pro surfers traveling the world in search of perfect waves. The cover says it all: "9 ISLANDS, 6 BOATS, 56 BIKINIS, 1 WETSUIT, 5 BROKEN BOARDS, 128 BARS OF WAX"!
- *Tropical Madness* (2001, Jet Girl Films). Shot by Australian filmmaker Lissa Ross and featuring more than fifteen of the world's top women surfers in exotic locations—but what sets this film apart are the candid interviews with the surfers.
- *Surf, Now* (2002, Roxy and Blue Field Entertainment). The first-ever girls' how-to-surf video—thirty-two minutes might not sound long enough to cover all the basics of surfing but *Surf, Now* comes close. Includes a brief history of surfing, and how to buy a surfboard, check the conditions, paddle out, turtle roll, and stand up. Great soundtrack and locations too.
- *Blue Crush* (2002, Universal Studios, now on VHS and DVD). The story of three surfer girls living on the North Shore of Hawaii. One of them, Anne Marie (Kate Bosworth) is training to compete in the Pipe Masters. Great footage of pro surfers Kate Skarratt, Rochelle Ballard, and Megan Abubo, with a cameo appearance by Layne Beachley. Best surf movie ever!
- *Heart of the Sea* (2002, Swell Cinema). A sixty-minute documentary celebrating the life of much-loved Hawaiian surfer Rell Sunn, who died of breast cancer in January 1998 (available online at www.swellcinema.com).
- *Poetic Silence* (2003, Billygoat Productions). An all-girl surf trip in the magical Mentawai Islands of Indonesia, featuring Rochelle Ballard, Megan Abubo, Serena Brooke, and friends.
- *The Modus Mix* (Billygoat Productions, VHS and DVD). The latest offering from the maker of *Poetic Silence*, *Peaches*, and the surf video *Blue Crush*. Each surfer girl featured—including Rochelle Ballard, Keala Kennelly, Megan Abubo, Lisa Andersen,

Holly Beck, Layne Beachley, and Kate Skarratt—stars in her own section, demonstrating her unique style.

● *Heart* (Andy Dangvu and Kassia Meador, DVD). Hot surfing by Kassia Meador, Prue Jeffries, Melissa Combo, Kim Wooldridge, and others, with a groovy sound track by Jamiroqai, John Butler Trio, Incubus, and Powderfinger. A surf movie with a difference.

● *The Surfers Journal Biography Series: Greats of Women's Surfing* (DVD). A look at the most influential female surfers of the twentieth century and beyond. Featuring Rell Sunn, Margo Oberg, Jericho Poppler, Lisa Andersen, Rochelle Ballard, Layne Beachley, Keala Kennelly, and others.

● *Angel Eyes, The Surfing Adventure* (Banzai Betty, VHS). Hawaiian surf movie featuring some of the most exciting surfers on the planet: Keala Kennelly, Layne Beachley, Megan Abubo, Trudy Todd, Jaqueline Silva, Rochelle Ballard, Prue Jeffries, Pauline Menczer, and Serena Brooke. As it says on the cover: It's rated E for epic!

● *The Road* (VHS). A road trip from Hawaii to Costa Rica, Australia, and California with the world's best women longboarders, including Julie Cox, Mary Bagalso, and Desire DeSoto.

● *One Winter's Day* (Frank Films, www.frankfilms.net). A thirty-minute documentary on one of the most inspiring big-wave surfers ever, Santa Cruz local Sarah Gerhardt who, in February 1999, became the first woman to surf Mavericks in Northern California.

● *Yoga for Surfers* (www.yogaforsurfers.com, VHS and DVD) A series of yoga clases designed by yoga instructor and surfer Peggy Hall to make you stronger and more flexible for surfing. Featuring pro surfers Rochelle Ballard, Taylor Knox, and Tom Carroll.

Also:

● *The Endless Summer* (1966, Bruce Brown). The first surf-trip movie, about two guys who travel the world in search of perfect waves. Features Pearl Turton, Australia's first surfing champion, surfing Palm Beach in Sydney.

● *Point Break* (1991). Hollywood movie about a bunch of surfing bank robbers. Keanu Reeves and Patrick Swayze are in it, but look out for the girl surfer called Tyler, played by Lori Petty—her stunt surfing was performed by former Australian pro-surfer Jodie Cooper.

● *The September Sessions* (2002, Jack Johnson). Okay, so it's not a girl's surfing video, but the fact that it's made by filmmaker/musician/surfer Jack Johnson should compensate for that. Plus, it features Kelly Slater, surfing and sharing some of his thoughts about the surfing life, as well as Rob Machado, Shane Dorian, Brad Gerlach, and Luke Egan.

Women's surfing magazines

SG
950 Calle Amanecer, Suite C
San Clemente, CA, 92673
Ph: (949) 492-7873
Fx: (949) 498-6485
E-mail: sgmag@primedia.com
www.sgmag.com

Surf Life for Women
3052 N. Main Street
Morro Bay, CA 93442
Ph: (805) 772-6896
E-mail: sunshine@surflifeforwomen.com
www.surflifeforwomen.com

Foam Magazine
Blue Water Publishing
P.O. Box 1338
Newport Beach, CA 92659
Ph: (949) 515-9270
www.foammagazine.com

Wahine Surfing
Online women's surfing magazine with news, contest results, a magazine section with articles (e.g., profiles of pro surfers, surf-fitness tips), details of upcoming women's surf camps and other events, a photo gallery, and links to surf-report sites.
www.wahinesurfing.com

Surfline Women
Surfline.com's women's channel, featuring women's surfing news, contest results from the tour, upcoming events, surfing tips from Layne Beachley and fellow pro-surfer Jodie Nelson, an online women's forum, surf travel stories (from pro surfers and readers), and video footage of women's surfing action.
www.surfline.com/womens

Other women's surfing websites

Bethany Hamilton Support Website
Bethany was attacked by a shark on October 31, 2003, while surfing near her home in Princeville, Kauai, with a friend. She survived the attack but lost her left arm just below the shoulder. Send her an e-mail, read about her accident, check out the photos of her surfing, and keep up-to-date with her contest results and surfing adventures.
www.bethanyhamilton.com

Blue Crush
A companion site to the 2002 Hollywood film, including surfing tips, a surf history timeline, an interactive surfing game to test your surfing knowledge, and a guide to the best surf spots.
www.bluecrush.com

Other surfing associations

Surfrider Foundation USA
The American branch (with over 37,000 members) of a global non-profit organization dedicated to the protection and enjoyment of the world's oceans and beaches.
P.O. Box 6010
San Clemente, CA 92674-6010
Ph: (949) 492-8170
Fx: (949) 492-8142
E-mail: info@surfrider.org
www.surfrider.org

Heal the Bay
A nonprofit organization established in 1985 to restore Santa Monica Bay, Southern California, to its natural, healthy state.
3220 Nebraska Avenue
Santa Monica, CA 90404
Ph: (310) 453-0395
Toll free: (800) HEAL-BAY (California only)
Fx: (310) 453-7927
www.healthebay.org

Surf Aid International USA

A nonprofit organization established to improve the health of the Mentawai people who live on the Indonesian islands that surfers visit in search of waves.
4660 La Jolla Village Drive, Suite 1040
San Diego, CA 92122
Ph: (858) 875-4581
E-mail: usa@surfaidinternational.org
www.surfaidinternational.org

Spirit of Surfing

www.spiritofsurfing.com.au
An Australian nonprofit organization that aims to promote goodwill and communication between surfers by encouraging them to respect the environment, surf breaks, and one another.

Surfers Code

Weatherproof metal plaques that are being installed at beaches all over the world explaining surfing's "rules of the road" in an effort to make surf breaks safer and less aggressive. To install a plaque at your local break, contact Miller Metal Imaging in Byron Bay, Australia, for the Surfers Code artwork: phone (612) 6685-5463 or info@millermetalimaging.com

The Kokua Hawaii Foundation

A nonprofit organization established in 2004 by surfer/musician Jack Johnson and his wife, Kim, to promote sustainable, environmentally friendly lifestyles through recycling, organic gardening, and eco-friendly art and music projects in elementary schools. "Kokua" is a Hawaiian word meaning "to help."
www.kokuahawaii.org

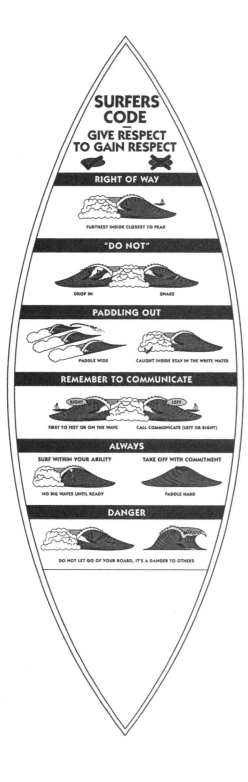

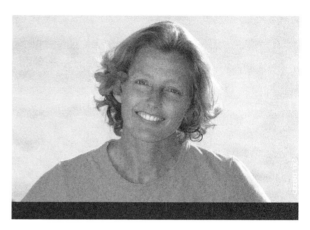

LOUISE SOUTHERDEN is a surfer, writer, and former editor of *Waves SurfGirl* magazine. Having lived the surfing lifestyle for more than twelve years and ridden waves all over Australia as well as overseas, she is now based on Sydney's northern beaches where she divides her time between her laptop and the waves.